THE
GREAT AMERICAN
HEALTH
HOAX

The Surprising Truth About How Modern Medicine
Keeps You Sick—How to Choose a Healthier,
Happier, and Disease-Free Life

RAYMOND FRANCIS

Health Communications, Inc.

D1115342

**Library of Congress Cataloging-in-Publication Data
is available through the Library of Congress**

© 2014 Raymond Francis

ISBN-13: 978-07573-1849-8 (Paperback)
ISBN-10: 07573-1849-5 (Paperback)
ISBN-13: 978-07573-1850-4 (ePub)
ISBN-10: 07573-1850-9 (ePub)

Publisher: Health Communications, Inc.
       3201 S.W. 15th Street
       Deerfield Beach, FL 33442–8190

Cover design by Larissa Hise Henoch
Interior design and formatting by Lawna Patterson Oldfield

CONTENTS

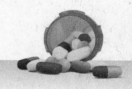

ACKNOWLEDGMENTS

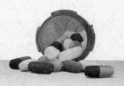

Many people helped in bringing this book to completion, and I would like to express to them my abundant and never-ending gratitude. First, I am grateful to the wonderful staff at my publisher, Health Communications Inc., and particularly to my editor, Allison Janse, for her many years of support, encouragement, and understanding.

I am also grateful to the unflagging support and excellent editing skills of Norman Hawker and Pamela Strong. Their dedication and willingness to work long hours on short notice helped to make this work a better, more readable, more useful book.

A huge debt also goes to my friends Richardine O'Brien, Mollie Meyers, Richard Higgins, and Joan Carole, who each contributed in their own way. I also want to thank Jeanelle Topping for her superior skills in organizing the bibliography.

Last, I would like to express my gratitude to the great thinkers who came before me and upon whose work I have built: pioneers such as Hippocrates, Claude Bernard, Antoine Bechamp, René Dubos, Alexis Carrel, Hans Selye, Walter Cannon, Otto Warburg, Linus Pauling, Roger Williams, Emanuel Cheraskin, Carl Pfeiffer, Russell Jaffe, Russell

Blaylock, and many others. I also want to thank my professors and colleagues at MIT who helped to sharpen the critical thinking skills that have helped me to achieve the insights that give value to my work.

INTRODUCTION

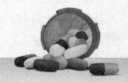

New opinions are always suspected,
and usually opposed, without any other reason
but because they are not already common.

—John Locke

There are three things which will bring
the end of civilization, even the mightiest that
have ever been or shall be ... impure water,
impure air, and impure food.

—Zend Avesta, 3000 BC

Health care in America is a hoax—it is pretending to be something it is not. This hoax is having a devastating impact on our health and quality of life, and it is threatening to destroy our economy and impoverish our people.

The definition of *health care* is "the maintenance or restoration of health." But our healthcare system is not about maintaining or restoring health—it's about managing the symptoms of disease. This is disease care, not health care! Managing the symptoms of disease does not prevent or cure disease. We need to transform to a true healthcare system, and it is up to you to help make that a reality.

Practitioners in our so-called healthcare system wait for disease to happen and then suppress the symptoms with toxic chemicals and invasive, health-damaging surgery. Because the underlying causes of ill health are not addressed, health is not maintained, people get sick and stay sick, and the costs skyrocket. Worse, the treatments themselves cause even more disease, pain, suffering, and death. You end up trading your original problem for a whole new set of problems. Instead of *maintaining or restoring health*, our healthcare system is a hoax that creates and perpetuates disease at enormous cost to society.

Most Americans today are trapped in a disease-care system that has little to do with health—or with science. We have been tricked into believing that disease care is health care and that chronic illnesses cannot be prevented or cured. This ineffective, expensive, and outmoded approach to health care must be discarded. Health is a choice, and you can learn how to choose it. The truth is that you can prevent or reverse almost any disease—without toxic drugs or surgery—by supporting the body's own innate ability to heal itself. To teach you what you need to know, this book offers a simple model of health that can empower almost anyone to get well, stay well, and never be sick again.

The Great American Health Hoax introduces you to a way of life that can become your highway to health. It will attempt to persuade you that you don't have to be sick. First, there is no fun in being sick, and second, we are going broke trying to pay for the cost of disease. As individuals and as a society, health is the solution. But it's a solution you must choose. After you decide to choose health, you have to learn how to achieve it. Fortunately, learning how to be healthy has never been easier. This book makes health simple.

By providing you with a simple road map to health, you *can* get well, stay well, and never be sick again. The goal is to educate a sufficient number of people like you so that we can put an end to our epidemic of chronic disease and provide a solution to the biggest social and economic problem of the twenty-first century—the problem of global aging.

The Problem

Global aging is the twenty-first century's major social and economic problem. By the year 2050, the number of old people will exceed the number of young people. In all human history, this has never happened before. The cost of providing pensions and disease care for the elderly is going to be astronomical, and there will not be enough young workers to pay the costs. This economic crisis is coming and unstoppable. We must act now to prepare. We cannot change the demographics, so the best solution is to reduce the need for care. Time is short, and the need is urgent.

The world is in the grip of a rapidly accelerating prevalence of chronic disease. This pandemic is killing us prematurely, lowering our quality of life, threatening our standard of living, and perhaps even threatening the future of our species. Our attempts to manage this problem through our current disease-care system are escalating the costs and presenting unprecedented political, moral, and economic dilemmas.

Ending this epidemic is a necessity. The alternative is to continue to choose disease, the consequences of which may be catastrophic. The rapid rise in chronic illnesses in children and adults is made worse by the fact that the number of older people is rapidly increasing. Disease-care costs are increasing and, even at present levels, are threatening to bankrupt the world's major economies, with the United States becoming like a third-world country, unable to pay its financial obligations. The resulting economic and financial meltdown will place unprecedented tax burdens on a shrinking working population and have a major effect on everything from our lifestyles to our political systems, and even our military security. Once this happens, daily life for most U.S. citizens will get dramatically worse.

For those who are retired or approaching retirement age, the available resources will not be sufficient to maintain the current level of benefits. This is one reason that learning how to stay healthy is so important. The National Institute on Retirement Security reports, "92 percent of working households do not meet conservative retirement savings targets for their age and income." Inadequate savings is a big problem for our older population. Rising disease-care costs along with fewer pension plans, stagnant home values, and low savings are a bad combination. Add to that the virtually certain reduction in the purchasing power of the dollar, and it gets worse. Uninsured health costs can be staggering, and more costs are being shifted to the individual at a time when incomes are not increasing. Since the cost of disease impoverishes the majority of older people, staying healthy is not just preferable; it is imperative. The cost of disease is the reason that the fastest-growing segment of the population filing for bankruptcy is age sixty-five and older. With increasing copayments and deductibles and reduction in covered benefits, this problem will only grow worse. To stay healthy, you must take personal responsibility and educate yourself on how not to get sick.

We have been mortgaging our future by spending money we don't have and making promises we can't keep. The U.S. Congressional Budget Office calls the path we are on *economically unsustainable*. Economists are telling us that the federal government needs to be making drastic changes in order to prepare for this time bomb threatening our future. Significantly increasing the retirement age, drastically increasing taxes, and reducing benefits have all been proposed. While they may be economically necessary, these changes are politically unpopular, so the government is paralyzed and nothing is being done to prepare for the grim realities facing us. So far, the solution has been to borrow money to pay the bills and then to print money and borrow more to pay off the loans. This approach has obvious limitations, with one of them being massive inflation that will reduce the standard of living for retired people and the middle class. Meanwhile, the problems mount daily without being addressed. The biggest danger is to continue to do nothing.

State governments have similar problems. The largest single item in most state budgets is Medicaid, in which costs have risen faster than tax revenues and are projected to rise even faster in the future. Like the federal government, states have been borrowing, and even selling assets, to pay for these bills. For example, Arizona sold its state capitol buildings. The cost of disease is forcing states to underfund the maintenance of roads, bridges, ports, education, and other investments that are necessary to foster future economic growth.

Economists say that the single largest drain on the economy is the cost of disease. Consider that the unfunded liabilities of Medicare are more than six times the unfunded liabilities of Social Security. Indeed, cutting the cost of disease in half could reduce our economic problems from unsustainable to manageable. This goal is worthy and achievable, but it cannot be attained by the current approach of more regulation and price controls.

Solving these problems urgently requires a new level of thinking. Instead, we are repeating the same old mistakes. Thus far, the public debate has been about how to pay for all this disease. Attempts to save a dime here and a dollar there are not the answer. The healthcare system requires transformational change to reduce the enormous waste caused by its inefficient and ineffective delivery system. This inefficient and ineffective system is why there are thirty-six modern countries that enjoy better health than Americans, at costs that are significantly less. Ultimately, the real solution, the win-win solution, is to teach people how to be healthy so that they don't get sick—*no disease, no costs*. Yet this solution, improving health, is not part of the debate. We need to change that. *We need to change the debate from how to pay for disease to how to prevent disease.* Better health must be seen as an achievable goal; it must become a priority. It must become *your* priority.

What we need is an educational campaign to teach people how to get well, stay well, and never be sick again. We need a true healthcare system that focuses on *maintaining and restoring health*. It can be done. Indeed, I have been doing this myself for thirty years, and many thousands have turned their health around by following the principles you will find in this book. Some say that because the subject of human health is so complex, it is impossible to teach people what they need to know to be healthy. Yet as Leonardo da Vinci once said, "Simplicity is the ultimate sophistication." We need to cut through the complexity and make health simple, so that even children can understand it.

The Solution

A sustainable society depends on the health of its citizens, and right now we have a sick population that is getting sicker with each passing year. To teach our population how to be healthy, a simple teaching tool is needed. The Beyond Health Model presented in this book is such a tool. It is fundamentally different and far more advanced than conventional medicine; it can take you beyond health as you know it. This model is based on the concept of One Disease, Two Causes, and Six Pathways to health and disease. It is a revolutionary concept offering the average person a simple guide for healthy living. It is science-based natural medicine, and it can give you the power to control your health in a way you never imagined possible. Contrast this with the unscientific, unnatural, ineffective, health-damaging, and very expensive system of medicine we have in place today.

The system of self-care presented in this book is based on a unified concept of how your body works, what goes wrong, and how to fix it. During the evolution of what we call "modern conventional medicine," there has never been such a framework tying everything together, which helps to explain why conventional medicine has been unable to prevent or cure disease; it lacks a scientifically valid theory of disease within which to operate. Scientific knowledge is increasing exponentially, yet medicine has consistently failed to incorporate new science into its clinical practice. As a result, conventional medicine is now so far behind the science and so deeply flawed that it is an impediment to progress—a major cause of disease and the leading cause of death—and is driving up the costs to unsustainable levels.

The truth is that we already know how to prevent and reverse almost all disease—no further research is required. There is no unavoidable reason that anyone should have heart disease, high blood pressure, cancer, diabetes, arthritis, Alzheimer's, osteoporosis, or any other chronic disease—or even suffer the occasional common cold. Health is a choice, and almost anyone can learn how to choose it. *You don't have to be sick.*

Have you ever thought about how wonderful it would be to live a long life, free of disease and disability? It's a great thought, isn't it? But how many of us think it is possible to do that? We can dream about it, but when we look around us, do we see it happening? Instead what we see is what is "normal" in our society. More than 75 percent of us have at least one diagnosable chronic disease. Whether it is allergies, autoimmune disease, clogged arteries, lung disease, or cancer, among people over age sixty-five, over 90 percent have these chronic diseases. Even our children are suffering an epidemic of ADHD, allergies, asthma, autism, cancer, diabetes, and obesity. Unfortunately, our own observations and experience lead us to believe that disease is inevitable, that we are not in control, and that good health and long life are the result of good genes or good luck—*but this is not true!* It really all depends on the choices we make.

Today, when it comes to health, as individuals and as a society, *we are doing most things wrong most of the time*, and it is making us sick and killing us. For example, the average American diet will not support healthy life—not even in rats. Yet we feed this diet to our children. We poison most of our water with fluoride and pollute the entire planet with tens of thousands of toxic man-made chemicals. Then we think of all the disease this creates as being normal.

What if we started doing most things right most of the time? Consistently choosing health-promoting, sustainable solutions will bring results that can seem like a miracle. You don't have to be a fanatic, and you don't have to be perfect. Just make the right choices most of the time instead of the wrong ones. Such changes require each of us to become educated and take personal responsibility for our health. The broader societal changes will require political leadership and support from business leaders, civic leaders, clergy, and educators. *But it all begins with you!*

Just because we are not all living long, disease-free lives now doesn't mean it's not possible. Many are doing it, so we know it's possible. It can become possible for you when you learn what it takes to be healthy and start applying that knowledge in your daily life. Given all the impediments to health today—such as our compromised food supply, toxic environment, electromagnetic pollution, unnatural lifestyles, and stressful lives—perhaps we cannot all achieve perfect health. But there is no question that we can do better than we are doing. It's relatively easy to live longer and healthier than your friends and neighbors. While they are struggling with heart disease, cancer, diabetes, arthritis, Alzheimer's, and hip replacements, you don't have to join them. Once you learn the true nature of disease, you will know what you need to do to attain superior health. In the following chapters I present you with cutting-edge science, translated into simple concepts, to empower you to achieve the health, vitality, and longevity that everyone would like to experience.

Unfortunately, the enormously profitable disease industry doesn't want you to know any of this life-saving information, and it does everything possible to obscure the truth. This science is not even taught in our medical schools; it is denied to our medical students who graduate woefully lacking in knowledge of nutrition, prevention, and wellness. Then, when bits and pieces of this science are presented to us in the media, the messages are often so confusing and contradictory that we don't know what to believe. Those who are invested in the status quo seek to create public doubt, even in the face of scientific consensus. The result is that very few of us are made aware of—let alone given the chance to benefit from—the priceless knowledge that could enable us to achieve long, disease-free lives.

The Reward

The key to success is simple. The human organism is a magnificent self-regulating, self-repairing system; it is capable of keeping you fully functional and in excellent health for well over 100 years of vital, productive life. Your job is to support this system. You are the sum of everything that goes into your body, which includes the nutrients, toxins, water, air, electromagnetic fields, thoughts, emotions, sunlight, and even noise. For the most part, you control what goes into your body. Given adequate support, your body will reward you with the gift of good health and long life. If we all did this, disease would all but disappear along with its costs, potentially preventing a catastrophic economic collapse.

All you have to do is take the knowledge we already have and put it to use. By making better choices daily, you will see the results for yourself. When you do this, you can end disease in your life. Not only will you and your family reap the benefits, but also you will be contributing to a healthier community, a safer country, and a saner world.

Health is a choice not yet chosen. To save ourselves and our economy, we must give health a chance. We need a tool to help us cut through the confusion and master the elements of health that are most important. This book is that tool. Come join me on a journey of learning and understanding that can empower you to get well and stay well. Choose health and never be sick again!

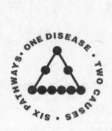

ONE

I Almost Died

There is no reason why human beings
should not reach the age of 150.

—Dr. Alexis Carrel,
Rockefeller Institute

The next major advance in the health of
the American people will be determined by what
the individual is willing to do for himself.

—John Knowles, former president,
Rockefeller Foundation

I f you want to choose health and get well, stay well, and never get sick again, this book will show you how. Human health is complex, but I have made it simple for you. Most of what is in this book I learned the hard way. That's why I want to make it easy for you. Knowing something about my ordeal will help you appreciate the science-based knowledge you will gain from this book.

People often ask me how I became interested in health. The answer is simple—I got sick and almost died. At the age of forty-eight, my death was a virtual certainty, and I came within inches of death from liver failure caused by prescription drugs. Needless to say, this experience focused my attention, and I became interested in health because I had to. Had I not learned what I needed to learn, I would almost certainly not be here, and you would not be reading this book.

I used my knowledge of biochemistry to save my life and to get well and stay well. Today, I am writing this book to share that knowledge, and I hope that once you learn it, you will share it with your family, friends, and neighbors. We need a revolution in how people think about health and disease, and you can be part of that revolution. Without it, we may be doomed to an economic catastrophe where the cost of disease will destroy our economy and impoverish our people. We all need to improve our health!

By learning the simple concepts I will teach you, you will achieve power over your health that you may never have dreamed possible. You will have the power to get well, stay well, and never get sick again. You will have the power to lose weight permanently, to prevent the common cold, to slow the aging process, and even to cure terminal cancer. That's a lot of power!

A good scientist never stops asking the question: Why? After restoring my health, I started to ask: Why did I get sick? Why does anyone get sick? How do you make a healthy person sick? If you become sick, how do you restore health? The answers to these questions started to come. They blew me away. It all made perfect sense, but nobody teaches us this stuff. It isn't even taught to our physicians.

My primary training is in chemistry. I am a graduate of MIT, but even with all my scientific knowledge, I still got sick and came close to death. Today, most people are getting sick and dying needlessly and prematurely because they don't know what to do to help themselves. Even worse, once you are sick, most of our physicians are of little help and too often do more harm than good. In fact, medical intervention is a major cause of disease and the leading cause of death in America.

We all would like to live a high-quality, disease-free life. But most of us have no idea of how to achieve that. We're not even sure it can be achieved. Our priorities get out of whack, and we form habits that jeopardize our health. We then ignore the early signs of ill health, and, without knowing it, we lay the groundwork for disaster. That is exactly what I did.

The early-warning signs that things were changing came in early 1983. I began to slow down, requiring more sleep and tiring more easily. I began to experience frequent allergic reactions, including runny nose, itchy eyes, sneezing, heart palpitations, and skin rashes. I suffered muscle aches and joint pain. I was losing the mental and physical capacity that had allowed me to operate at the highest levels of international business and government. Life was becoming more like a chore.

I brought these complaints to the attention of my physician, a professor at Harvard Medical School. He examined me and did thousands of dollars worth of testing. The tests all came back normal, and he pronounced me in "excellent health." When I protested, saying I did not feel like I was in excellent health, he replied, "You are getting older." When I said that in my whole life I had never felt this way before, he said, "You have never been this old before." I was forty-six years old.

The truth is that my health was already seriously compromised, and this man's ignorance was astonishing, especially given his exalted position as a professor of medicine at a prestigious medical school. Yet this level of ignorance is what we teach in our medical schools.

I was complaining of fatigue. Fatigue is the number-one complaint that doctors hear, yet my fatigue was attributed to my "advanced age" of forty-six. The truth is that age has nothing to do with fatigue. I am now seventy-eight, and I have boundless energy. Fatigue is the result of disease. As we start to get sick, one of the first things to go is our ability to make or use the high-energy compounds that energize our bodies. Everything in your body runs on energy, and unless you have abundant energy, you are already seriously ill. Without energy, nothing will work right. You are sick! The fact that I was fatigued should have been ringing alarm bells. The doctor should have sprung into action to find the causes of my problems, correct them, and restore me to good health.

Unfortunately, looking for causes is not the way our physicians are taught to think, and they have no protocols or established procedures for measuring early decline in health. Instead they blame "getting older" for so many feelings of ill health, even at ages when human beings have the potential to be in their prime. Physicians consistently assume that the patient is "well" until his or her condition deteriorates into symptoms that the doctor recognizes as a diagnosable disease. In truth, by the time you have a so-called diagnosable disease, you are *really* sick.

Over the next year and a half, my symptoms worsened. My fatigue became more pronounced; I required ever-increasing amounts of sleep, and even then I felt tired. The fatigue made it increasingly difficult to travel, which my job as a management consultant required. My allergic reactions were becoming more severe. I would experience sneezing fits so dramatic that I would have to rest after them. Heart palpitations were frequent and pronounced. I would see colored rings around lights and my vision would blur.

Because of my allergic reactions, I decided to seek the assistance of an allergist. Little did I realize as I entered the physician's office that it would be the last day of life as I had known it. The allergist administered a diagnostic test called an *intradermal* test, whereby an allergen is injected into the skin. Intradermal tests are more sensitive and may identify allergies that the typical scratch tests might miss. The doctor neglected to tell me that the FDA regularly received reports of injuries and deaths from these tests. My overall condition should have prompted this physician to be more cautious and anticipate that an intradermal test might provoke a serious reaction.

It did.

The reaction was catastrophic, causing my immune system to spin out of control. During the next week I slept constantly and appeared to have aged about ten years. I suffered fatigue and disability unlike anything I had ever experienced. Prior to the test, despite some fatigue and allergy problems, I was still able to function normally. After the test, I was completely dysfunctional, unable to perform any meaningful activity.

Years later, another physician—one considerably more intelligent and better informed—described how my state of compromised health and immunity was like standing on the edge of a cliff. The allergist should have recognized my vulnerability and the need to work initially with nutritional support and conservative treatments to back me away from that edge. Instead, his decision to administer a provocative test pushed me off the cliff and into an abyss of catastrophic health decline.

Ten months later, I was still in that abyss with my health in a downward spiral. In the past, whenever I had been sick, I had always recovered quickly. This time was different. I experienced chronic fatigue, multiple chemical sensitivities, and allergic reactions to almost everything. I also developed autoimmune syndromes, including Sjogren's syndrome, Hashimoto's thyroiditis, and lupus. In these syndromes, the immune system attacks the body's own tissues, causing a cascade of serious problems. In my case, my immune system was attacking my salivary glands, lachrymal glands, thyroid gland, kidneys, and connective tissue. I suffered from fibromyalgia and had an extensive list of debilitating symptoms, including dizziness, memory loss, depression, heart palpitations, blurred vision, muscle and joint pain, diarrhea, bloating, nausea, numbness, and seizures. I suffered grand mal seizures so severe, they would propel me out of a chair and onto the floor. I was unable to perform any meaningful activity. My health was gone, and life as I had known it was over.

During those ten nightmarish months, I visited thirty-six top specialists. I had so many different symptoms that I was referred to specialists for each one, including ophthalmologists, gastroenterologists, neurologists, endocrinologists, cardiologists, allergists, rheumatologists, psychiatrists, internists, and immunologists. Being bounced from one specialist to another was very frustrating. Even worse, it was useless. My multitude of symptoms totally baffled those learned experts. How much easier it would have been had they known what I know: that there is only one disease and that *symptoms are not important.*

These physicians performed many expensive diagnostic tests, which served little purpose other than to give fancy names to my symptoms, such as arrhythmia, arthralgia, colitis, keratitis sicca, neuropathy, thyroiditis, lupus, and others. They spent a small fortune so that they could describe my symptoms with technical names, the usual diagnosing—then sent a bill. Not one of them had a helpful suggestion! Not one of them had even the slightest understanding of what was wrong. A few suggested that I was a hypochondriac, imagining ill health, and referred me to psychiatrists. The psychiatrists couldn't find anything wrong, so they referred me back to the referring physician. It was a frustrating and expensive merry-go-round.

Many physicians assume that if they don't know what's wrong then the patient must be crazy. They blame the patient, not their own ignorance. Back in the 1980s, chemical sensitivities and chronic fatigue were considered mystery diseases, and most patients were referred to psychiatrists. These syndromes are now more accepted as legitimate because so many people have developed them. At the time, I thought my doctors were baffled because my case was so complex. In the end, the answers proved to be simple, one just needed to look for them.

From Bad to Worse

As sick as I was after ten months of illness, things were about to become *much* worse. One of the last physicians I went to see made a decision that nearly killed me. He prescribed an antibiotic called metronidazole, which is known to be toxic to the liver. Given my condition, my liver was already under a lot of stress; it was unable to handle the additional toxic load. My liver failed, and I was at death's door. I would later learn from the medical literature that I should have never been prescribed such a drug. I should have known better, given my prior experiences, but trusting the doctor, I took the drug.

As I lay in bed, dying of chemical hepatitis, my weight dropped from an already trim 160 pounds (at six-feet-two) to a positively skeletal 120. I was too weak even to lift my head from the pillow. My vital signs were failing rapidly, and my physicians said there was nothing they could do.

Had I continued to rely on conventional (allopathic) medicine, I certainly would have died, but I didn't know where to turn for help. As I look back, I am amazed at the chain of events that saved my life and allowed me to restore my health. My brother started the process. He gave me a book that proved instrumental in saving my life: Norman Cousins's bestseller, *Anatomy of an Illness*. In 1964 Norman Cousins, a layman with no medical or scientific training, was diagnosed with ankylosing spondylitis, a connective tissue disease that deteriorates collagen (the "glue" that holds our cells together). Cousins's disease was literally causing his body to fall apart. His illness, like mine, was deemed by his physicians to be incurable and fatal. Unwilling to accept such a prognosis, Cousins sought whatever knowledge he could to help himself. He succeeded.

Cousins took action in four areas. First, like myself, Cousins recognized that medical treatment was harming him. He concluded that the drugs his physicians were prescribing were so toxic that they were accelerating his decline. He stopped taking the drugs. Second, he discovered the enormous power of the mind over the body. The excruciating pain he was experiencing was affected by his attitude toward the pain. By learning to change his attitude, he could reduce his pain. Third, he found laughter to be helpful; ten minutes of genuine, hearty laughter would cause his pain to go away for hours. He started watching funny movies, and when the effect would wear off, he would switch on the projector and laugh some more. The laughter had profound and beneficial effects on his body chemistry and contributed to his recovery. Fourth, he discovered the powerful anti-inflammatory properties of vitamin C. He decided to take twenty-five grams a day administered by intravenous drip. This action had a profoundly beneficial effect on his highly inflammatory condition. By avoiding toxic prescription drugs, changing his attitude, laughing, and administering plenty of vitamin C, Cousins saved his life and made a miraculous recovery.

I wondered how Cousins managed to find the pertinent information he needed to save himself. If Cousins, a dying man with no scientific training, could obtain such critical, life-saving knowledge, why couldn't his physicians? Instead, they were doing him more harm than good!

Knowing that Cousins had found a way to save his own life encouraged me; I hoped that my scientific training as a chemist might enable me to do the same.

As I lay there with a poisoned liver, dying from chemical hepatitis, I realized that if I wanted to live I must act quickly. Thinking about how instrumental vitamin C was in Cousins's recovery, I recalled that vitamin C plays an essential role in liver detoxification. Because my liver had been poisoned by a toxic drug, perhaps some vitamin C would help. It seemed like an experiment worth doing.

It worked!

Within two days after starting oral doses of vitamin C (about 4 grams a day), my vital signs were stabilizing and I was able to sit up in bed. A few days before, death had been a certainty. Now I could sit up, which was the first time I had experienced a measurable improvement in all those months. Progress, even in the form of something as simple as sitting up in bed, can be incredibly inspiring. At that point, I knew I could take action that would make a difference. Meanwhile, my physicians could not understand why I was still alive and actually improving.

Still alive, but a frail skeleton. I had difficulty performing the simplest tasks, such as dressing or tying my shoelaces. I had no energy and became fatigued from the slightest exertion. My hands and feet were numb; I had difficulty walking and moved slowly. I was lightheaded and tended to fall over easily. Worse, my brain wasn't functioning; I felt like I was in a mental fog. I had difficulty with short-term memory and simple calculations. Even as I improved enough to venture out again, I easily forgot where I was going or what I intended to do. I would purchase groceries and then drive home, leaving the groceries in the store.

Perhaps worst of all was the extreme chemical sensitivity that I continued to suffer. My body was no longer able to safely process common environmental chemicals. The smallest amount of exposure to man-made chemicals would cause me to become debilitated. When I turned on a water faucet, the subtle chlorine fumes coming out with the water were enough to cause me to become weak, lightheaded, and disoriented. I could not read or be near printed materials because of the chemical fumes coming from the ink and paper. I used only a speakerphone because I would react to the fumes outgassing from the plastic telephone receiver. My gas water heater had to be replaced with an electric unit because I reacted to the combustion fumes diffusing into the surrounding living space. I had to wear clothes made only from natural fibers to avoid the toxic fumes from synthetics, with polyester being the worst of all. I had to purchase special water and air filters. But even with these many precautions, the relentless reactions to environmental chemicals were a living nightmare.

Someone who has not personally experienced chemical sensitivity has great difficulty understanding how just a whiff of certain chemicals can create total, debilitating havoc in a matter of seconds. I remember taking a small piece of Scotch tape off a roll and being devastated for the rest of the day by the seemingly inconsequential chemical odor from the tape. With chemical sensitivity, the nervous system develops a memory of past reactions. Upon detecting these reactive agents again, even in infinitesimal quantities, a full-scale response occurs. Our modern world is permeated with chemicals that can produce such reactions in susceptible people.

In this hideous state of health, I fell into a deep depression. I thought about taking my life. Although I had made a small amount of progress, I was allergic to almost everything, and I was in a constant state of debilitating reactions. My life was ruined. No doctor could help me. I was unable to do any meaningful activity and had nothing to look forward to. I could not even watch television because of the chemical fumes outgassing from the TV set as it heated up.

Choosing to Live

One beautiful afternoon, I was sitting out in the sun and contemplating the meaning of life. Illness has a powerful way of providing perspective and time to think about the really important things. I asked myself whether I wanted to continue living. After some long deliberation, I decided that I did not want to die. I wanted to live. However, life was not worth living in such a debilitated state. My only option was to find a way to restore my health.

How could I do this? My doctors could not help. In fact, they were mostly responsible for my sorry state. I recall thinking about the explosion of knowledge in the world—about all the new scientific data being published every day. I thought that if we had the technology to send men to the moon, then surely, somewhere, there must be some key bit of information that could help me. I became determined to find out whatever I could. It was not easy. My vision was blurred and my eyes were in pain. Given that I was unable to be near printed materials because of the ink fumes, how could I study? My mind didn't work right either. In my early quests to research my health condition, I would find myself lost in a mental fog, spending hours reading the same material over and over without realizing it. Ironically, I was reacting to the very materials I was using to learn how to restore my health.

Still, I remained determined. I purchased a respirator mask to protect me from the chemicals coming from the ink in my study materials. Unfortunately, the rubber part of the mask gave off toxic fumes. I took the mask apart, boiled the rubber pieces in water for two days and then reassembled it, which made the mask tolerable so that I could wear it while I did the necessary work. Next, I purchased a portable electric oven and one hundred feet of outdoor extension cord. I placed the oven downwind from my house and baked all of my reading materials in order to drive off the ink chemicals. Bizarre, but it worked. Now at least I could handle and read my rapidly accumulating piles of medical and scientific literature. I began to educate myself, looking for clues that might help to restore and improve my health. Thus began a new phase of my life, which continues to this day.

As I searched for solutions to my problems, I read technical papers written by a biochemist who, like me, had become chemically hypersensitive. No physician had been able to help him either. His sensitivity was so great that he was forced to leave his family and move to a small wooden shack on a remote beach to get away from man-made chemicals. Eventually, through his understanding of biochemistry, he was able to restore his health and function normally once again.

Knowing that someone else had been able to heal himself of this horrendous condition gave me the hope I so much needed. His example convinced me that I, too, would be able to help myself to understand the chemistry of my illness and apply sound scientific principles to solve my problems. It took me two years of learning and experimenting to raise myself from the depths of liver failure, chronic fatigue, autoimmune diseases, and chemical hypersensitivity. Recovery required a great deal of persistence, willingness to try new things, and acceptance of many setbacks. In particular, I had to be extremely careful about the products I selected. Even minute amounts of toxins were enough to make me very ill. I ended up with a kitchen full of vitamin supplements that I could not take because of their toxic impurities and my level of susceptibility to them. I now know that even healthy people are harmed by these impurities; it is just not evident to them.

I learned the hard way how suffering can come when health is failing, and when you try remedies that do more harm than good. Even with my scientific training, finding the answers was difficult. Particularly with vitamin supplements and personal care products, a great deal of conflicting information abounds, and consumers remain confused about how to make the best choices. Accurate health information is in great demand, and that is precisely what this book provides for you.

I was able to return to work in late 1987, but I became increasingly focused on the problems of disease in our society. In July 1991 I resigned from all my business and community activities, including all the boards I served on, deciding to devote myself to teaching others how to be healthy. I started by speaking to groups—at first, the same support groups to which I had belonged during the depths of my illness. Then I branched out to a wider audience, which evolved into a regular evening workshop series that continued for more than a decade. A publisher became aware of my work and invited me to write a column for his newspaper. I started a syndicated radio show that I hosted for sixteen years, providing health information for all who wanted to listen. I began publishing my own newsletter, *Beyond Health News*, and then writing a series of books, one of which you are now reading. Because of my bad experience with vitamin products that contained impurities, I started my own vitamin company, Beyond Health International (see Appendix A). I make sure that Beyond Health manufactures only the purest and highest-quality vitamins possible, and in biological forms that maximize their metabolic activity in the body. Making products of extraordinary quality requires extra knowledge, care, and cost, which is why only a handful of suppliers do this. The final results are more than worth the effort.

Reaching Our Potential

One of the most profound conclusions I have reached is that health is a choice, but it's a choice we aren't choosing. The potential for human health and longevity is far greater than we are now achieving. Studies describe populations who lived longer and healthier lives than we do, simply because their societies made dietary and lifestyle choices that supported human health. With just a little knowledge and effort, we can do the same. We can choose health, but first we must educate ourselves.

My own quest for an understanding of how the body maintains and heals itself continues to this day. Throughout my research, I continue to ask myself basic questions, such as:

- What is health?
- What is disease?
- How do people get sick?
- How can disease be prevented or reversed?
- How long can people live in good health, and what does it take to achieve this?
- What is the potential for human health and longevity?

Answering these questions has enabled me to develop a revolutionary concept of health and disease—one that is so simple and yet so powerful, it gives you the power of choice to never get sick again. Please allow me to teach you how your body works and how you get sick. Once you know this, you are in control, which benefits you and your loved ones, as well as society as a whole, by reducing the costs of disease.

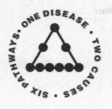

TWO

Why It Isn't Working

*There is no reason in the world why over 75 percent
of the American people should be suffering from
degenerative and deficiency diseases. Disease never comes
without a cause. If a person is sick and ailing it is because
he has been doing something wrong. He needs an
education in how to live a healthy life.*

—Jay M. Hoffman, Ph.D., *Hunza*

*Each person carries his own doctor inside him.
They come to us not knowing that truth. We are at
our best when we give the doctor who resides
in each patient a chance to go to work.*

—Dr. Albert Schweitzer

T he human body is designed to be healthy. So why are we
experiencing an epidemic of chronic, degenerative disease
and going broke trying to pay for it? Despite the trillions of dollars

we have spent on medical research and health care, the incidence of chronic disease continues to increase. The body has built-in mechanisms to repair damage, optimize performance, and keep you fully functional—well into your hundreds. So why isn't this happening? The truth is that our epidemic of chronic diseases, such as heart disease, cancer, diabetes, osteoporosis, arthritis, and Alzheimer's, is something we have created by making mistakes. There is no excuse to continue to make these mistakes. *We created this epidemic—we can uncreate it!*

The Changes We Have Made

Never before in human history have so many health-related factors changed so rapidly and so completely. The basic nutritional, environmental, and behavioral dimensions of human existence have been altered severely and rapidly. Since the Industrial Revolution, and most especially during the past century, we have:

- Completely changed our diet.
- Created a toxic environment.
- Developed new patterns of behavior and lifestyle.

You cannot make so many fundamental changes and expect them to have no effect. We are now experiencing the results of these changes. Our way of life is completely different from the lives of even a century ago. In terms of a human life span, these changes have been made too slowly for us to notice, but from an evolutionary standpoint, they have come too rapidly for healthy adaptation by our bodies and minds.

Granted, in this millennium, most of us cannot grow our own food and harvest it when ripe, walk to our destinations, and avoid all the stresses of modern industrial society. However, by recognizing what contributed to the health of traditionally healthy people, combined with an understanding of the significant changes we have made to our own environments and lifestyles, we can learn how to compensate. We can learn how to make healthy choices while still living a modern way of life.

Here are some examples of how we are creating our problems and making ourselves sick.

Changes to Our Diet

- Fruit and vegetable plants are now grown with artificial fertilizers that produce more food per acre, but these foods are deficient in essential nutrients. Modern farming methods have led to depletion of minerals in the soil, which leads to mineral deficiency in us.
- Many foods are harvested before they are ripe to prevent spoilage during transportation and distribution. Premature harvesting does not allow food to reach its full nutritional maturity.
- The nutritional content of food deteriorates during storage, transportation, and distribution. Nutrition starts declining within hours of harvesting. In two days, the losses are significant, yet the average age of produce in a supermarket is two weeks. The average age of apples is ten months.
- Most of our food is processed in order to make it easier to store and consume. Processing depletes the nutritional content. Such foods include sugar, flour, pasta, bread, breakfast cereal, and other canned, bottled, and packaged foods.
- Cooked foods are also nutritionally inferior to raw ones, and most of the American diet consists of both processed and cooked foods.

Changes to Our Environment

- The farming of large single crops has created new and serious problems of insect infestations, creating the need for insecticides. Insecticides, along with the use of herbicides and fungicides, have made food production methods a significant contributor to our toxic environment and toxic food supply.

- The modern processed-food industry adds man-made preservatives, flavors, colors, and other toxic chemicals to our foods. No one knows what the combination of all these chemicals is doing to our bodies.

- Energy production from coal, oil, and gas is constantly polluting our environment.

- Virtually all of our industrial processes—from printing our daily newspapers to painting our homes and building cars and computers— have led to the introduction of thousands of man-made chemicals into our environment. These chemicals put toxic loads into our bodies, disrupt hormones, and interfere with neuroimmune defense and repair systems. Of the 100,000 chemicals in commerce today, barely 4,000 have been tested for safety and only a few dozen for interactive effects. Meanwhile, about 4,000 new chemicals are added each year.

- Electromagnetic pollution is damaging our health, but we aren't paying attention because we can't see it, smell it, or feel it.

Changes in Our Behavior and Lifestyle

- Movement is essential to health and life itself, yet we are the most sedentary people in history.

- Sunlight is like an essential nutrient, but most of us live and work indoors and don't get enough.

- The body has its own biological clock that is essential to health. Our nocturnal lifestyles are upsetting that clock.

- The constant noise in our society is not only damaging our hearing, it is upsetting our normal biochemistry.

- Man-made sources of radiation, such as x-rays, are damaging our genes.

- Stressful lifestyles, with demands for performance run by the clock, are taking a toll.

An editorial by Joseph Scherger, M.D., in a 2000 *Hippocrates* edition said, "Lifestyle factors now loom as the leading cause of premature death."

Most people expect to be sick at least one or more times each year, to have to cope with at least one serious illness by midlife, and in all likelihood, to die of one or several diseases by their eighties, if not sooner. Most people also think that poor health is mainly the result of bad luck or bad genes and that good health and longevity are a matter of good fortune. Nothing could be further from the truth.

With few exceptions, poor health is a matter of choice. But most of the time, we don't know we are choosing to be sick because no one ever told us that. If someone did tell us, we didn't believe it; our health-nut cousin told us not to eat sugar, but what did she know? Unfortunately, many young people today are sick because of the poor choices that their parents and even grandparents made. Disease is not like a meteorite falling out of the sky and hitting us over the head. We make ourselves sick by making bad choices. Conversely, we get healthy and stay healthy by making good choices.

Most people think that they are healthy as long as they are able to function normally. Few people know what optimal health actually feels like. This level of health, with its disease-free boundless energy, vitality, and mental clarity, is rarely experienced in our modern, industrialized society. Perhaps that's why hardly anyone accepts the notion that a vigorous and healthy life beyond 100 years is within reach. In reality, that kind of long, healthy life is what we should all expect. We know this because communities of people around the world have traditionally achieved this level of health.

A Poor Record

Very few of us are growing old in good health and dying naturally of old age. Instead, we get sick and die from entirely preventable diseases such as cancer, heart disease, stroke, Alzheimer's, and diabetes.

The United States spends far more on health, in total and per capita, than any other nation. Yet the World Health Organization ranks the United States only thirty-seventh in overall health. Given that the United States spends more than anyone else, shouldn't it be the healthiest nation on Earth? Do you suppose the fact that the Standard American Diet will not support healthy life, even in rats, could be a factor?

People in their teens or early twenties should be at peak levels of health, but that's not what's happening. The majority of our young people are sick with allergies, asthma, attention deficit, autism, cancer, diabetes, obesity, and other diseases. Autopsies performed on accident victims of this age group reveal that nearly 80 percent have early stages of heart disease, and 15 percent have arteries that are more than half blocked. These young people thought they were healthy; they appeared to be healthy; they lived normal lives; but they were definitely not healthy.

Immigrants to the United States are, on average, healthier and live longer than the general population, largely because they tend to adhere to their traditional diets. The second generation, however, tends to adopt the processed-food American diet, and their health suffers.

It's a matter of perspective. Our own ill health does not stand out when compared to our unhealthy friends and neighbors. The allergies, the colds, the flu, the arthritis, the premature aging—all of these seem perfectly normal. Because disease is so common, we have come to believe that it is an inevitable, natural, normal part of the aging process. We mistake being able to function for being healthy. We perceive "sick" as being bedridden or housebound, and "healthy" as being able to go about our normal activities. But being healthy is far more than being free of obvious disease symptoms. Healthy means that all of your cells are functioning at the highest level that genetic capacity allows. Ask yourself: Are you truly healthy with all of your cells and systems working as they should, or are you just not obviously sick?

Unfortunately, we are a sick population, growing sicker by the day and, worse yet, blind to our sickness. Here are some realities:

- More than three out of four Americans have a diagnosable chronic disease.
- More than two out of three regularly take prescription or over-the-counter drugs.
- More than three out of four people over age sixty regularly take two or more prescription drugs.
- One out of four children under age eighteen already has at least one chronic disease.

Despite all this, two out of three Americans believe themselves to be in "good" or "excellent" health. How can you think you are in good or excellent health when you are taking medications and experiencing symptoms of disease? It's because disease is so common; we think disease is health so long as we can keep functioning. As long as we continue to think that disease is health, improving health becomes difficult. If you lack vitality or have other bothersome symptoms, you are not healthy, and if you have a diagnosable disease, you are definitely not healthy.

For example, most people with allergies don't think of themselves as having a chronic immune dysfunction disease; they think of allergies as an inconvenience in an otherwise healthy body. But chronic allergic reactions accelerate the aging process, tax the body and the immune system, and make you much more susceptible to infections and other diseases. Allergies are not just a benign inconvenience; they are a serious immune disorder. Every allergic reaction does long-term damage to the body, reducing longevity. Healthy people do not have allergies.

We are in a state of denial. Some people assert that we are now healthier and living longer, but that claim is medical industry propaganda. The incidence of virtually every chronic disease continues to increase, and the health of the American people is in a long-term downtrend.

The Colossal Failure of Modern Medicine

Our epidemic of chronic disease is the result of the fundamental changes we have made in our diet, environment, and lifestyle, but another dimension to our problems is the colossal failure of conventional medicine to provide meaningful health care. In fact, medical intervention has become the leading cause of death in the United States.

Conventional medicine excels at trauma care and crisis intervention. However, that is only 10 to 15 percent of medicine. The other 85 to 90 percent doesn't work. It is completely inadequate for dealing with chronic and degenerative disease because it has little to no basis in science. It doesn't even meet the basic requirements of logic and common sense in the light of what is known scientifically. For chronic conditions, conventional medicine is not only ineffective, it does more harm than good.

We teach our medical students to look at symptoms, give the symptoms a name, and then prescribe drugs to treat that so-called disease. These students learn nothing about health. Health is rarely even mentioned in most medical schools. Nor are they taught to look for or address the underlying causes of the problem being presented. Yet only by addressing causes can problems be solved. Treating symptoms with drugs solves nothing; it only makes the disease chronic and creates a host of new problems. New problems arise because prescription drugs work by poisoning the body. Drugs are toxins that block enzymes and receptors. They do nothing to cure disease; they merely suppress the symptoms, while their toxicity creates havoc, throwing the body's chemistry into chaos.

Biochemical chaos is disease, and prescription drugs cause chaos. This is why medical intervention is a leading cause of disease and the leading cause of death. To obscure these inconvenient facts and the entirely new disease problems caused by drugs, our physicians don't call these new problems "diseases"; they call them "side effects." When you are sick, your body chemistry is abnormal. The only way to restore health is to restore normal chemistry. Drugs do exactly the opposite; their toxicity creates even more abnormalities and disease. To base an entire medical system on the use of toxic chemicals will go down in history as one of humankind's greatest blunders.

Most people think of conventional medicine as the best that our science has to offer. Wrong! The real problem with medicine, and the reason it is so dysfunctional and dangerous and inflicts so much needless suffering, is because it has little basis in science. Everyone who has studied this matter has arrived at similar conclusions: about 85 percent of all medical procedures have no basis in science. Based on anecdotal evidence, they have never been proven by scientific method to be safe or effective.

We have the technology to travel to Mars, yet we have a system of medicine that is stuck in the seventeenth century. The origin of conventional medicine's problems can be traced back to Isaac Newton and the seventeenth-century philosophers and scientists who saw the universe as a giant machine. As a result, physicians began to look at the human body as a machine, a grouping of separate parts and pieces, similar to a mechanical clock. By contrast, much older traditional Chinese medicine looks at the body as a complex energy system, with disease as disharmony in the system. This difference is critical because the body is not just a bunch of parts stuck together. You cannot treat one part and expect success.

It is astounding that while almost every other human endeavor, whether in the sciences, business, economics, or investment, has advanced to a whole-systems approach, medicine is stuck focusing on the parts. Disease is viewed as symptoms limited to a body part, separate from the body as a whole. The physician's job is to treat the symptoms. But suppressing symptoms is not the same as eliminating the systemic causes of the symptoms. This mechanical view of the body works well if you have a broken bone. However, it doesn't work at all if you have cancer or some other systemic disease. This is why data from the National Center for Health Statistics show that the cancer survival rate today is essentially the same as it was in 1950. No progress has been made, and no progress can be made as long as the focus remains on the tumor, the part, while ignoring the systemic process that created the tumor.

Meanwhile, modern science recognizes the body as a complex energy system and disease as an imbalance in the system. In fact, the human body is a battery-operated electronic device—far from a mechanical clock. Yet conventional medicine remains stuck in a mechanistic view. This is why, with each passing year, conventional medicine falls further behind the science, becoming more and more expensive, impotent, and irrelevant. In 2001 the National Academy of Sciences issued a report concluding that conventional medicine is now so far behind the science, it is no longer possible to bring it up to date. Conventional allopathic medicine needs to be discarded, and we need to start over with a new systems approach—one that focuses on the body as an energy system.

The Web of Life

Choosing health would be easy if only one factor were involved. However, no one factor determines our health. Rather, our state of health is the result of countless biological and behavioral interrelationships called the "web of life." Unwittingly, we have been busy pulling this web apart through the fundamental changes we have made in our diet, our environment, and our lifestyle. Everything relates to everything else; making a change in one part of the web affects the rest of it.

We are learning that the systems that support life are more interdependent and delicately balanced than we ever realized. The web is as big and complex as the planet itself. No one fully understands how it all works. But the fact that we do not understand it thoroughly should not prevent us from using what we do know to protect and support our health right now.

Our health is deteriorating because we have screwed up big time. If you want to achieve a high level of health in today's world, you need knowledge, commitment, and a willingness to make new choices. It can be done. None of us can revert to the life of our primitive ancestors, even if we wanted to, but you can, with a few changes in your diet and lifestyle, improve your health and quality of life. You just have to know what changes to make; you will learn what these are in the following chapters. Embracing the principles presented in this book will not only directly benefit you and your family, it will also help others wake up from a pharmacological trance and loosen the economic stranglehold of a failed healthcare system.

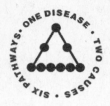

THREE

Making Health Simple

Simplicity is the ultimate sophistication.

—Leonardo da Vinci

*The specific disease doctrine is the grand
refuge of weak, uncultured, unstable minds. . . .
There are no specific diseases.*

—Florence Nightingale

Conventional medicine is obsessed with giving groups of symptoms different names, which is why we have over 12,000 different diseases. The result is massive confusion and powerlessness in the face of so much complexity. Many people end up lost and bewildered, unaware that they have the power to cure themselves. This is why we need to simplify.

Conventional medicine focuses on suppressing symptoms. This approach to disease causes diseases to become chronic, health to deteriorate, and costs to skyrocket. In this chapter, you will learn a new approach. This new way of thinking about health and disease employs a model that recognizes not thousands of diseases but only one disease, with just two causes. This simple model enables you to address those two causes, empowering you to prevent and cure almost any disease. This model is so powerful that it can take you beyond health as you know it, so that you never have to be sick again.

Seeking Simplicity—Removing the Mystery

At the time of my near-fatal illness, I probably knew as little about disease as most people. I thought disease was something that happened to the unlucky, the starving, or those who really abused themselves, such as alcoholics and drug addicts. My scientific education suggested that disease came from germs and genetic predisposition. My physician told me that my problems were the result of getting older—as opposed to choices I had unknowingly made and could choose to reverse.

During my recovery I realized that I could have prevented my problems if I had understood what causes disease. I recognized that as long as disease remained mysterious and difficult to understand, then only the high priests of medicine—the educated experts we call doctors—would be able to deal with it. But in truth, they can't deal with it any better than you can. They don't understand what causes disease and certainly don't know how to cure it. I began to wonder: What if we could *all* understand what causes disease? Wouldn't that empower us to prevent disease, and by addressing the causes, even cure it?

To most of us, disease is a mystery, one that can be very frightening. In the face of serious disease, we feel powerless, so we outsource our health to the experts. However, even those with a thorough knowledge of germs, genes, medicines, and surgery cannot prevent and cure disease.

Learning more about these complex subjects would thus not help people take care of themselves. What we need are solutions that take the mystery out of disease, so that ordinary people can put them to use.

One of the great scientific minds of the twentieth century, biochemist and Nobel laureate Dr. Roger Williams, wrote that cells malfunction and die for two reasons: "First, because they do not get everything they need; second, because they get poisoned by something they decidedly do not need." Dr. Williams is saying that we can live long and healthy lives if we do two things right. One is to provide our cells with all the nutrients they need. The other is to protect our cells from toxins. To the extent that we can accomplish these tasks well, we can prevent disease and extend the length and quality of our lives.

If all your cells are working the way they should, you cannot be sick. When a sufficient number of cells malfunction, internal communications and self-regulation systems become destabilized, resulting in biochemical chaos. This chaos increases the number of compromised cells, causing a downward spiral that leads to the disabling of critical defense and repair mechanisms and to diagnosable disease. By the time the first signs of disease become noticeable, normal cell function has already been compromised significantly. Fatigue, aches, pains, skin problems, frequent colds, sinus problems, digestive problems, allergies, and any number of other symptoms all indicate massive cellular malfunction.

Contrary to popular opinion, germs do not cause disease. Unless you experience massive exposure, you have to already be sick or injured in order to develop an infection. In other words, only sick people get sick. Otherwise, everybody who is exposed to a given "bug" would become sick, and this is not the case. No question, an infection makes you even sicker, but contrary to the common notion that we "catch" infectious diseases, an infection indicates that cellular malfunction had already weakened the immune system. Having a cold or the flu is like a warning light on your car's dashboard. Unfortunately, few of us pay attention to these alarms. We think that getting a cold or flu is normal, and that once the symptoms are gone we are well again. Not so. Healthy people do not get infections.

We live in a society that does not have an accurate understanding of disease, nor of what is required to create and maintain health. As members of a society where more than three out of four of us have a diagnosable chronic disease, our view of health is distorted. Most of us are sick, yet we tend to think of ourselves as in good or excellent health. When symptoms of disease appear, we are surprised and often feel like helpless victims, as if struck by lightning. You need to remember the following:

Abnormalities in the body's chemistry cause disease. Restoring this chemistry to normal cures disease. Keeping this chemistry normal prevents disease.

There Is Only One Disease: Malfunctioning Cells

How is this for simplicity? *There is only one disease.* Once you understand there is only one disease, it takes the complexity out of disease. *This simple concept of* one disease *puts the power over disease into your hands.*

What is this one disease? *Malfunctioning cells.* A cell is a microscopic unit of life, and each of us starts life as a single cell in our mothers. That one cell grows into a community of tens of trillions of cells communicating and cooperating with each other—we call this community our *bodies.* All tissues and organs are made of cells; all bodily functions are carried out by cells, and these cells are specialized depending on the function they perform. *Your cells are what make your life possible.*

Understand what your cells need, what causes them to malfunction, and you will have the knowledge you need to get well and stay well.

When your cells are functioning normally, they communicate with each other to keep your biochemistry in balance, and your body is self-regulating and self-repairing. This balanced state is called *homeostasis*. When you are in homeostasis, your body regulates its internal conditions, regardless of outside conditions. A simple example of homeostasis is the body's ability to maintain its internal temperature within a narrow range, despite large variations in the outside temperature. When cells malfunction and the body's abilities to communicate, self-regulate, and self-repair are impaired, the body goes out of balance; we call this *disease*.

We put a lot of wear and tear on the body every day. If your body is not fully self-repairing daily, repair deficits accumulate, and your body will soon let you know. Any illness is a sign that you need repairs that your body isn't making because your cells are deficient and toxic. If you don't keep up the maintenance on your car, repair deficits make it age, break down, and end up in a junkyard. Your body is no different. Repair deficits manifest as aging, disease, and disability; people with large repair deficits end up sick, frail, and in nursing homes, unable to care for themselves. People line up for hip replacements and knee surgery because their joints are wearing out; their bodies are falling apart from lack of repair. In fact, all chronic disease involves repair deficits, which is why they are degenerative. Whichever disease label your physician has pasted on you, whether it is arthritis, allergies, diabetes, cancer, Alzheimer's, or osteoporosis, all are due to cellular malfunction and repair deficits.

As part of the body's normal maintenance and repair process, old cells are constantly replaced with new ones. The body produces hundreds of billions of new cells every day. If new cells are not constructed with proper building materials, they will be unhealthy and weak, yet most of us are deficient in at least several essential nutrients. Without the necessary building materials, cells are unable to perform their normal tasks, including routine repairs. Tissues made from such cells are inherently vulnerable to sickness and injury. Ultimately, the body's self-regulation systems break down. Due to the poor diets and the toxic environment in our society, cells are often deficient and toxic when first created, becoming progressively more so over time. This situation is precarious, with a large number of cells either malfunctioning or functioning at a borderline level. Similar to walking a tightrope, falling off is easy. Because your reserves have been depleted, any number of stressful factors can derail you, be it an emotional event, a pathogenic organism, a night out on the town, a physical injury, or even a lengthy airplane flight. Almost any challenge to a compromised system can be the straw that breaks the camel's back. To get well and become biologically younger, your job is to make every new cell better than the one it's replacing.

Invariably, people suffering from disease have made poor choices (if unknowingly) and caused their own illness. In the case of sick children, the parents have made the poor choices. We are not taught to take responsibility and make better choices about our health. Instead, when we become sick, we look to something outside of ourselves to explain our misfortune. We prefer to think of disease as something that happens to us, as if randomly falling out of the sky. By placing the blame for sickness on factors outside our control, we relieve ourselves of responsibility.

Getting well involves shifting the body back into normal repair mode. To do this, you have to give your cells all the materials they need by eating a good diet and taking high-quality supplements, *and* you must keep your cells free of toxins that can interfere with your repair machinery. When you do this successfully, your body will once again properly communicate, self-regulate, and self-repair, and homeostasis will be restored. You will become biologically younger, mentally sharper, stronger, healthier, happier, and disease free. If you are sick, it's because you are not treating your cells properly.

Once you understand the concept of malfunctioning cells and only one disease, you'll see that all the thousands of so-called diseases do not exist. So if they don't exist, why does diabetes look different from Alzheimer's and heart disease look different from cancer? It's because the cellular malfunction manifests in different tissues due to a specific combination of deficiencies and toxicities acting through a unique set of genes. *In every case, all symptoms result from cellular malfunction.*

Alzheimer's disease is the symptom of cells malfunctioning in the memory part of the brain. Parkinson's disease is the symptom of cells malfunctioning in the motor part of the brain. Macular degeneration is the symptom of cells malfunctioning in the optic nerve. Breast cancer is the symptom of cells malfunctioning in the breast. Arthritis is the symptom of cells malfunctioning in the joints. In each case, we have cells malfunctioning in a different part of the body, but to think of them as different diseases is self-defeating and indicates a lack of understanding of the true nature of disease. To empower ourselves to prevent and reverse *all* disease, we need to focus on what is common to each disease, not on what is different.

Common to all disease is cellular malfunction. Either your cells are functioning as they should or they are not. It's that simple. If they are not functioning as they should, you can exhibit thousands of symptoms in different body parts. Our physicians call them thousands of diseases, but if cells were not malfunctioning, there would be no symptoms. *No matter what the symptoms, if you restore cells to normal function, the symptoms go away.*

For example, what we call "cancer" is cells that are growing uncontrollably because their communication and growth control mechanisms are malfunctioning. When cells malfunction, depending on a number of factors, including your unique genetic makeup, different symptoms occur. To give different names to different symptoms may be useful for discussion purposes, but counterproductive for treatment purposes. *The name of your disease doesn't matter, because there is only one disease and only one treatment.*

You can call certain symptoms "cancer" if you like, but how does that help you? Does it tell you how you got the cancer? Does it tell you how to prevent cancer or how to cure cancer? Don't be confused by the name. Once you know that cancer is cellular malfunction, the issue becomes simple. Now you know what it is, why you got it, and how to prevent and reverse it.

To prevent disease, prevent cellular malfunction. To reverse disease, restore malfunctioning cells to normal. These statements hold no matter what your disease is called.

There Are Only Two Causes of Disease: Deficiency and Toxicity

To restore cells to normal and reverse disease, you have to address why the cells are malfunctioning. *There are only two causes of cellular malfunction, and therefore, only two causes of disease: deficiency and toxicity.* Cells are either getting too little of what they need or too much of something they don't need. Disease is the effect of deficiency and toxicity, and to cure any disease, you must focus on addressing the two causes of disease.

Are you having a problem embracing this simplicity? Are you asking, "Doesn't chronic stress cause disease?" Yes, it does, but through the same two causes—deficiency and toxicity. Manufacturing stress chemicals depletes the body of critical nutrients, causing deficiency, and the buildup of stress chemicals has a toxic effect on the body. Even infectious and genetic diseases manifest because of deficiency and toxicity. A bacterial infection harms you by using precious nutrients, causing deficiency, and also by producing toxins that poison the body. When genes malfunction, they are not producing what they should be producing (deficiency) or are producing too much of something they should not be producing (toxicity). In every case, it always comes back to deficiency and toxicity—the two causes common to all disease.

Think of each single cell in your body as a vast industrial park containing thousands of factories, producing tens of thousands of life-sustaining chemicals every day. Some of these chemicals are hormones to help regulate your body; some are neurotransmitters to enable you to learn, think, and remember; and some are antibodies to keep you free of infection. Each cell contains hundreds of powerhouses, called *mitochondria*, to produce the energy of life. There are also warehouses, a central computer, traffic directors, communications systems, raw-material delivery systems, waste disposal systems, security systems, and much more. All of this metabolic machinery knows how to function perfectly if the right raw materials are available, toxins are not interfering with normal operations, and the operating instructions have not been compromised. In each cell, every second, there are about 100,000 chemical reactions taking place with literally trillions of individual activities occurring. Our job is to support all this. When we don't, we get sick.

A chronic deficiency of even one nutrient will make you sick. The average American is chronically deficient in at least several essential nutrients.

We know that even one toxin can disable critical metabolic machinery or give incorrect instructions to the machinery, creating chaos in the cells and the body. The average American is in toxic overload, with hundreds of toxins accumulating in their tissues. Our out-of-control epidemic of chronic disease is the direct result. To end the disease epidemic, we must start a revolution to end deficiency and toxicity. This revolution can begin with you.

Suppose you go to your doctor with the following three complaints: asthma, arthritis, and depression. The doctor examines you and determines that you also have high blood pressure and osteoporosis. According to conventional medicine, you now have five diagnosable diseases and will probably be referred to several specialists. Perhaps you will see a pulmonary specialist for your asthma, a psychiatrist for your depression, and a rheumatologist for your osteoporosis. You will definitely be prescribed drugs: perhaps a bronchodilator and a corticosteroid for your asthma, acetaminophen for your arthritis, several drugs for your hypertension, Fosamax for your osteoporosis, and Prozac for your depression. None of these drugs will cure you. On the contrary, the combination of them will be so toxic that you are guaranteed to develop entirely new disease problems, but these will be called "side effects" so as not to alarm you. Additional drugs may be prescribed to suppress the symptoms of these newly created problems, but since drugs are toxins, the more drugs you take, the sicker you will get.

In the case above, you are being treated incorrectly for five diseases, when in reality, you have only one disease, and that disease needs to be cured—not treated. What you have is a large number of malfunctioning cells, and even though you have multiple symptoms, these could all be stemming from one cause. Mercury, for example, is a toxic heavy metal that, even at extremely low doses, can cause all of the above so-called diseases, at the same time, in the same person. Sources of mercury include dental amalgam fillings, vaccinations, and seafood. Careful removal of the mercury fillings by a specially trained dentist, avoidance of vaccinations and seafood, and chelating supplements to remove heavy metals are ways to eliminate the true cause, rather than treat the various symptoms. Once you do this, all five "diseases" will disappear. This option is far better than taking toxic drugs to treat them, which not only keeps you sick but makes you even sicker.

Just as one toxin like mercury can cause a number of so-called diseases, *a deficiency of even one nutrient can cause a similar list of diseases.* For example, a deficiency of vitamin D can cause many diseases, including asthma, cancer, and osteoporosis. The prostate gland is a zinc-rich tissue; a zinc deficiency will cause prostate problems. The thyroid gland is an iodine-rich tissue; an iodine deficiency will cause thyroid problems. The cervix is a vitamin C– and folate-rich tissue; women with low vitamin C have a 1,000 percent increase in cervical cancer risk. Thousands of so-called diseases can result from deficiencies, and you can be sure that conventional medicine will treat almost all of them incorrectly because our physicians have not been trained to understand this: *There is only one disease and only two causes of disease: deficiency and toxicity.*

Cells malfunction only if they suffer from a lack of nutrients (deficiency) or an excess of something not needed (toxicity), and usually a combination both. Because most of us are chronically deficient in several essential nutrients and are accumulating hundreds of toxins, experiencing an epidemic of chronic disease that is out of control should not be a surprise. You have the power to prevent these two causes of disease because you are able to choose how you live your life. All you have to do is give your cells what they need and protect them from what they don't need.

Six Pathways to Health or Disease

Your health is a continuum from perfect homeostasis on one end to terminal illness on the other. At any moment, one of two things is happening: you are either moving toward better health or toward more disease. Almost all of us, whether we have any serious complaints or not, are somewhere between perfect health and terminal illness and moving toward disease. We must turn this around and move toward health.

Think of it this way: Imagine two cities—Health and Disease. Six major highways connect these two cities. If you are traveling on all major highways toward Health, you will end up in Health. On the other hand, if you are traveling toward Disease on all the highways, you will end up in Disease. Most Americans are heading toward Disease because they don't know any better, but you don't have to be one of them. We all make daily choices that determine where we are on each pathway, in which direction we are heading, and how fast we are going. Get yourself moving toward health on all Six Pathways and you will remain biologically young, healthy, and vigorous. We do not know all of the many factors that could be affecting your health, which is why using all six of the pathways at the same time is important. In this way, you can be confident that you are addressing a broad spectrum of potential causes for your problem.

The Six Pathways are:

1) Nutrition
2) Toxin
3) Mental
4) Physical
5) Genetic
6) Medical

A holistic approach to health requires attention to all of these pathways. Consistent movement in the wrong direction along any of them can lead to the breakdown of self-regulation and self-repair and the cellular malfunction that is disease. Continuous movement in the right direction leads to optimal health and performance. The body knows how to take care of itself, provided you give it what it needs to do so. Good choices along each of the Six Pathways will provide for the needs of your body just as sunshine, water, and rich soil provide for the needs of a houseplant. It isn't complicated; in fact, it's incredibly simple. We just get lost along the way because we don't have a roadmap. Well, now we do have such a roadmap: One Disease, Two Causes, Six Pathways. I call this the Beyond Health model. Applying this model can help you to restore balance to your cells and support your cells' natural ability to regulate and repair. Along each of the Six Pathways I will teach you how to prevent the two causes of disease—what it takes to restore health and prevent future sickness. The following chapters address how you can get yourself moving in the right direction on each pathway.

Most people continue to believe that disease is the result of bad genes and bad luck, and that diagnosis with a chronic disease means long-term treatment with expensive drugs, a lower quality of life, and often death without dignity. All this changes once you know how your body works and how you get sick. Now you are in control. Giving your cells what they need and protecting them from harm is the key to health, and this is something you can do yourself.

Accepting responsibility for your health can be enormously empowering, but you need knowledge and tools to do this. Educate yourself and learn how to make healthful choices that will lower your levels of deficiency and toxicity, and promote your cellular health. *The overall health of our cells—determined by relative levels of deficiency and toxicity—is the sole determinant of our health.*

To help you master your health and make it simple, in the next chapter I have provided a list of maintenance items that demand your attention. The good news is if you get yourself moving in the right direction on each of the Six Pathways, this maintenance will happen automatically.

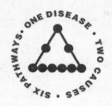

FOUR

Your Maintenance List

My approach is to start from the
straightforward principle that our body is a machine . . .
and it can be subjected to maintenance and repair
in the same way as a simple machine, like a car.

—Aubrey de Grey, Ph.D.

A living cell requires energy not only for all its functions,
but also for the maintenance of its structure.

—Albert Szent-Gyorgyi, M.D., Ph.D.

Human health is almost infinitely complex. That's why to end our epidemic of chronic disease the focus needs to be on simple, practical steps that anyone can take to optimize health. This chapter presents a list of maintenance items that are fundamental to your biochemistry and your health. Learning to maintain and control them will reduce your risk of developing disease and, if you are already sick, will help you to get well and stay well. Performing this maintenance will even reverse some of your aging and make you biologically younger.

A car that is not well maintained ends up in a junkyard. A body that is not well maintained ends up in a nursing home. Nobody wants to end up in a nursing home or be dependent on others for basic needs, with a quality of life that is close to zero. Yet one out of seven people over age sixty-five suffer from chronic conditions that impair their ability to live independently. A car that is 100 years old can still look and run like new if it is well maintained, and so can you, if you are well maintained. Here is the problem: We don't know how to maintain ourselves.

Cars come supplied with an owner's manual and a maintenance schedule that tells you what to do to keep the car in good running condition. We don't. With cars, most of us know we need to change the engine oil, keep the tires inflated, rotate the tires, replace the radiator fluid, change the brake and transmission fluids, replace the timing belt, replace the brake pads, replace hoses and filters, and numerous other maintenance items, especially as the car becomes older. How many of us know how to maintain a human body?

If you don't keep a car well maintained, you may be in for some expensive problems. You may end up needing a new engine, radiator, or transmission. Likewise, if your body is not properly maintained, you may be paying for a $40,000 hip replacement, a $50,000 knee replacement, $100,000 open-heart surgery, or well over $100,000 for cancer treatment. It's cheaper to do the maintenance and avoid these problems. Regular preventive maintenance can extend the life of your vehicle, and it can extend your life, too.

Below is a list of maintenance items that require your attention. If you perform this maintenance, you can move yourself toward health by keeping your body machinery in top operating condition. This will extend your life and allow you to live those extra years filled with vitality and free of disease. These maintenance items are as follows:

- Energy production
- Inflammation
- Acid/alkaline balance
- Digestive health
- Hormonal balance
- Platelet stickiness
- Fat storage

Energy Production

The amount of energy you are able to produce may be the most important measure of your health. Virtually all chronic disease involves impaired energy production. Everything runs on energy, including you. When your energy is high, you are healthy. When it's low, you are sick. When it's very low, you are very sick. When it's gone, so are you. Optimize your energy production and you optimize your health, longevity, and quality of life.

A decrease in energy production is an alarm that things are seriously wrong. Yet low energy is epidemic, and fatigue is the number-one complaint made to doctors. Fatigue was the first complaint I brought to my doctor when I began my downward health spiral. I told him I didn't have the energy I used to have. After a comprehensive and expensive examination, my doctor, who was a Harvard Medical School professor, joyfully announced that all of my tests showed that I was in excellent health and that my fatigue was the result of getting older. Like most physicians, this professor of medicine was clueless that decreased energy production was a serious matter, and that my lack of energy was not about getting older. It was about being very sick. Healthy people have boundless energy. Any decrease means you are sick, and decreased energy often occurs long before other symptoms of disease. Think of a healthy college athlete. That's high energy. That's where we should all be.

Every cell contains hundreds to thousands of energy production units called *mitochondria*. Like the engine in your car, mitochondria produce energy by reacting fuel with oxygen. Most of the energy is in the form of heat to keep your body warm, but mitochondria also produce chemicals that the body uses for energy, such as the high-energy compound adenosine triphosphate (ATP). Anything that interferes with the production of ATP will cause fatigue. The ability to produce high-energy compounds is very much affected by deficiency and toxicity. For example, niacin (vitamin B3) is used in the creation of energy; a niacin deficiency results in less energy. A deficiency of essential fatty acids impairs the ability to properly construct mitochondrial membranes. Improperly constructed membranes result in progressive loss of energy production and disease. Toxic metals like mercury can disable enzymes required for energy production. Prescription drugs and environmental toxins like herbicides and pesticides can impair ATP production. Consuming the food preservative sulfite can cut ATP production in half.

Maintaining high energy levels is critical to your health. Less energy means less ability to deliver nutrients and remove toxins, and less ability to do daily repairs to DNA and tissues. Shortness of breath is often an indicator of energy production problems. How many of us feel winded walking up several flights of stairs? How about running up those same stairs? How many people have a problem exerting themselves much at all? How many are barely sustaining life? In order to be truly healthy, you have to optimize your energy production.

Fructose presents a special problem. Metabolizing fructose drains ATP from cells, robbing the body of energy. Our overconsumption of fructose is causing myriad health problems, including loss of energy, high blood pressure, diabetes, excess uric acid production (gout), and chronic inflammation. Inflammation, which we'll talk about soon, causes damage to DNA, mitochondria, and tissues throughout the body. The largest source of this vicious cycle is the habit of drinking sodas containing high-fructose corn syrup.

So-called diseases of aging, such as Alzheimer's, cancer, and diabetes, are all related to decreased energy production. Energy is required for every bodily function, and less energy reduces the body's ability to remove toxins and do its daily DNA and tissue repairs. Today, our energy requirements are higher because of all the environmental chemicals our bodies are being forced to detoxify. We must be careful to avoid toxins that interfere with energy production, such as heavy metals and pesticides. *We must supplement with nutrients such as the B vitamins; vitamins C, D, and E; CoQ10; acetyl L-carnitine; alpha-lipoic acid; curcumin; essential fatty acids; ribose; and phospholipids that help to increase energy production.*

How can you gauge how well you're doing on this maintenance item? It is possible to measure your energy production by using a technique called bioenergy testing. But the simplest way is by noticing how you feel. When you wake up in the morning, do you bounce out of bed ready and even eager to begin your day? Everyone needs periods of rest and relaxation, but is your energy sustained and dependable throughout the day and evening? Do you enjoy daily moderate exercise and occasional strenuous exercise?

If your answer to some or all of these questions is "no," remember, it's not because you're getting older. It's because of deficiency (one or more things are missing) and toxicity (one or more things are gumming up the works). The solution to your personal energy crisis is a unique combination of factors. You will find these solutions in the following chapters on the Six Pathways.

Inflammation

Inflammation, when needed, is a good thing. It is the body's natural and healthy response to injury, irritation, or infection. If you cut your finger, an inflammatory process begins immediately; this is what causes redness and swelling. The inflammatory process neutralizes harmful microorganisms, helps to repair the wound, and cleans up the debris resulting from the injury.

Temporary inflammation is beneficial, but chronic inflammation is disastrous. Chronic inflammation destroys your body! During the normal inflammatory process, white blood cells destroy harmful microorganisms by unleashing powerful chemicals called *free radicals*. These free radicals can potentially go on to damage healthy tissue, and even DNA. However, once a repair has been made, the inflammatory process is turned off, and the free radicals it has generated are subdued and neutralized by chemicals called *antioxidants*.

However, when inflammation is turned on and not turned off, a constant supply of free radicals is generated that overwhelms your antioxidant reserves. The resulting damage to tissue and DNA ages you and causes disease of every description. For example, most hip replacements are necessitated by inflammatory damage to the joint. A better idea is to protect the joint from inflammation, keep it in good repair, and it will last a lifetime—surgery unnecessary.

Unfortunately, chronic systemic inflammation is epidemic. Why? Because our diet, environment, and lifestyle promote inflammation. The average American's diet is rich in pro-inflammatory factors, including sugar, wheat, and excess omega-6 fatty acids. At the same time, it lacks antioxidant and other anti-inflammatory nutrients found especially in fruits and vegetables. Consuming an acidic diet containing too much salt, sugar, white flour, dairy, meat, and cola drinks also contributes to inflammation. Many experts consider overacidity to be one of the major causes of chronic inflammation. Being overweight makes things worse because fat cells produce inflammatory chemicals. Environmental toxins have an inflammatory effect and deplete antioxidants. Taking antibiotics leads to chronic gastrointestinal inflammation. Chronic stress produces hormones that result in chronic inflammation. People who are sleep deprived have higher levels of inflammation. Even chronic noise causes inflammation.

Inflammation is a common element in virtually all disease. Most of us are suffering from some degree of chronic low-grade inflammation, and many suffer from severe inflammation. No matter what so-called disease you have, from cancer to the common cold, inflammation is a major part of your problem. By promoting chronic inflammation we are aging ourselves prematurely, causing us to look old, feel tired, and suffer every imaginable disease. Learning how to reduce inflammation will go a long way toward preventing and reversing almost all disease as well as slowing the aging process, keeping you healthy, biologically young, and vigorous for a lifetime. To be healthy, you must eliminate or at least minimize chronic inflammation.

The amount of inflammation in your body is a powerful predictor of aging, age-related disease, and whether you will become fragile in old age. Russell Tracy, Ph.D., professor of pathology and biochemistry at the University of Vermont College of Medicine, helped demonstrate that inflammation is the cause of heart disease. Dr. Tracy maintains, "Inflammatory factors predict virtually all bad [health] outcomes in humans."

In Alzheimer's patients, the areas of the brain clogged with senility-associated plaques also bristle with inflammatory cells and cytokines (cytokines are proteins released by cells that trigger inflammation). Research has found that cytokines block memory formation in mice. In diabetes, inflammation and insulin resistance track together. Inflammation is also a culprit in declining lung function, osteoporosis, and old-age depression. Inflammatory activity breaks down skeletal muscle, leading to the loss of lean muscle mass.

Inflammation also contributes to the shortening of telomeres. Telomeres are caps at the ends of chromosomes found in each cell. Like the plastic tips on shoestrings, telomeres protect the ends of the chromosome strands. Telomere shortening is a marker of aging and disease.

Inflammation is easy to see if you cut your finger, and it's easy to feel if you pull a muscle. But chronic inflammation can smolder on for years without symptoms. Eventually, you may experience aches, pains, and soreness. But because inflammation can be silent, it is useful to measure your levels with blood tests like *C-reactive protein* (CRP), *interleukin 6* (IL-6), *plasma viscosity* (PV), *and erythrocyte sedimentation rate* (ESR).

Learning how to live an anti-inflammatory lifestyle is a key to your health and longevity. Controlling chronic inflammation requires a comprehensive approach because it arises from a combination of causes, but most of it is under your control. In the chapters on the Six Pathways, you will learn how to prevent and control inflammation. Supplementing with antioxidant nutrients is essential to control chronic inflammation and restore health. People with serious illness may require massive amounts of antioxidants to shut the inflammation down. These include omega-3 fatty acids; vitamins A, C, D, and E; beta-carotene; CoQ10; curcumin; quercitin; selenium; N-acetylcysteine; and alpha-lipoic acid. Taking a high-quality vitamin C to bowel tolerance (just short of the amount that causes loose stools) is recommended. The B vitamin complex (including folate, B6, and B12) is also critical to controlling inflammation. Dietary restriction inhibits the inflammatory response, which explains why low-calorie diets promote longevity.

Acid/Alkaline Balance

The pH of your cells and body fluids has a major effect on your health. pH is a measure of the acidity or alkalinity of a solution. Aqueous solutions with a pH less than 7 are acidic (think vinegar), 7 is defined as neutral (like water), and greater than 7 is alkaline (think lye). pH controls an enormous amount of body chemistry. *If your pH is wrong, your chemistry will be wrong, and nothing will be right!*

To function normally and keep your body in homeostasis, your cells need a proper environment. Internal temperature, glucose levels, oxygen levels, sodium levels, and pH must be kept within normal limits. The pH of the fluid inside a healthy cell is between 7.35 and 7.45, which is slightly alkaline. Maintaining normal pH in your cells and tissues is one of the most important things you can do for your health. Maintaining normal pH is not optional—you must do it! Fortunately, this is something you can measure yourself and control.

One reason that pH is so important is the regulatory functions that protein molecules perform. Special protein molecules perform critical metabolic and regulatory functions to keep your body functioning and balanced. The success of these functions depends on the protein maintaining the correct geometric shape. Changing the shape of the proteins damages your metabolic machinery and impairs your ability to self-regulate and be healthy. *The shape of the proteins can be altered by even the tiniest changes in pH!*

When your pH is normal, you will slow the aging process, have more energy, and be healthier. When your pH is not normal, cells malfunction and you are sick—even if you don't think you are. Too many people suffer from the delusion that they are healthy, when actually they are already sick and getting sicker because their pH is declining. When they finally arrive at a diagnosable disease, such as cancer, they are usually surprised and don't realize how long it took them to get there.

Tragically, our physicians have little understanding of the true causes of disease and will usually blame your problems on getting older or on faulty genes, when the real problem is your declining pH, which has nothing to do with age or genes. Virtually all degenerative diseases, including arthritis, cancer, gallstones, heart disease, kidney stones, osteoporosis, and tooth decay, are associated with excess acidity.

How Do Our Bodies Become Acidic?

Although normal cell metabolism produces acids, a healthy diet rich in alkalizing minerals can neutralize these acids. However, abnormal cell metabolism is another matter; it produces enormous amounts of acid, which is the major reason that so many of us are too acidic. Normal cells produce energy through a process called oxygen respiration, where fuel (mostly fats and some glucose) reacts with oxygen. However, our poor diets, accumulation of toxins, and lack of exercise all conspire to impair the ability of our cells to produce energy through oxygen respiration. When this happens, cells switch to a less complex, less efficient way of producing energy called fermentation. Fermentation produces lots of lactic acid and free radicals. Free radicals must be neutralized with anti-oxidants, but due to the lack of antioxidants in our diet, these radicals cause systemic inflammation. Lactic acid can be neutralized by alkaline minerals, but modern diets are deficient in alkalizing minerals, so our bodies build up lactic acid and become too acidic.

The shift from normal oxygen respiration to fermentation is a major factor in accelerating the aging process and is associated with numerous diseases, especially cancer. In fact, the prime cause of cancer is loss of 60 percent or more of a cell's oxygen respiration capacity. (See my book *Never Fear Cancer Again*.)

Making matters worse, we consume too many acid-forming foods such as sugar, highly acidic cola drinks, excess salt, grains, dairy, and meat. On average, Americans eat far too much animal protein. When animal proteins break down in the body, they metabolize into strong acids. The bottom line is that the majority of the foods most of us eat today have an acidic effect on the body. As a result, most of us suffer from chronic low-grade acidosis, which leads to chronic inflammation. Chronic stress creates acidity, and we lead stressful lives. Allergic reactions create acidity, and most of us have allergies and food sensitivities, whether we know it or not. Chronic dehydration, chronic infections, most prescription drugs, and many environmental toxins all promote acidity.

To stay healthy, the body must neutralize excess acids, and healthy bodies have alkaline reserves that can be used for this purpose. However, when fermentation and our acid-forming diets deplete those reserves, the body starts taking alkalizing calcium and magnesium from the bones, resulting in osteoporosis. Acidosis also increases the production of free radicals, which damage DNA, cause disease, and accelerate the aging process. Even a small amount of acidity can lead to fatigue and feeling generally subpar. Pain is a symptom of acidity. Acidity can even make you fat. Acidic cells have a lower metabolic rate, preventing fat from being burned.

Low pH and Enzymes

Abnormal cellular pH impairs the function of enzymes. Enzymes are little molecular machines that put molecules together or take them apart. Critical chemical reactions in the body are completely dependent on enzymes. Digesting food requires enzymes to take molecules apart, and making complex molecules like hormones or neurotransmitters requires enzymes to put them together. However, enzymes are pH sensitive. Change the pH and you change enzyme function, potentially shutting down critical metabolic machinery. For example, the liver's ability to detoxify and to produce hormones is dependent on pH-sensitive enzymes. When the pH is abnormal, liver detoxification is compromised; hormones may become unbalanced; immunity will be depressed; food may not be properly digested; chemicals critical to brain function may not be produced. The pH in a cell gives chemical signals to genes, instructing them to perform or not perform certain actions. Abnormal pH will give abnormal instructions to your genes, causing cells to malfunction and make you sick.

Low pH and Cellular Oxygen

The body must be slightly alkaline in order for your cells to be properly oxygenated. A slightly alkaline solution can absorb more than 100 times as much oxygen as a slightly acidic solution. This is why when cellular pH drops, oxygen levels drop, causing a host of problems. Acidic body fluids will not support the oxygen-rich environment that the body needs; this can manifest as chronic pain, impaired metabolism, infections, and cancer. When the fluid inside and outside the cells becomes too acidic, cell walls begin to lose their integrity. This not only damages the ability to transport oxygen into cells, it also allows toxins to enter cells. These toxins can damage DNA, causing mutations that further compromise a cell's ability to fight off disease. Viruses and bacteria normally living in your body, without causing harm, will suddenly be activated in a low-oxygen environment, causing infection. Our physicians then blame the "germs" and give us antibiotics, instead of normalizing our pH.

It's All About Energy

Beyond acidity and alkalinity, pH has another critical dimension in the realm of energy. While most of us don't think of it this way, the body is a battery-powered electronic device. Each cell is a little battery, and because pH is actually a measure of voltage, your cellular pH reflects the strength of your batteries. Remember this about your batteries:

- When your batteries are strong, you are strong and healthy.
- When your batteries are weak, you get tired and sick.
- When your batteries are very weak, you are seriously ill.
- When your batteries are dead, so are you.

To be healthy, you must keep your batteries fully charged. Electricity plays an enormous role in almost every function in the body. One example is your heart. Physicians measure the electrical activity in the heart with a test called an electrocardiogram. Electricity generated by your cell batteries signals the heart to beat; weak batteries cause problems with your heartbeat. Many heart patients have been given pacemakers, surgically implanted commercial batteries, to treat abnormal heart rhythms. A far better alternative is to strengthen your electrical system and use your own batteries as Mother Nature intended—surgery not required. Medicine in the future will be focused more on the body's electronics and energy systems. Fortunately, you don't have to wait for the future; you can take care of your electronics now by paying attention to your pH.

Like any electrical device, the body is designed to run at a certain voltage. Cells operate normally at a voltage of -20 to -25 millivolts (mV). There is a direct correspondence between the voltage and the pH of your cells. A voltage of -20 mV corresponds to a pH of 7.35, and -25 mV corresponds to a pH of 7.45. The minus sign in front of the voltage number means that the system is electron giving, which indicates your batteries are strong. This is what you want in order to be healthy. On the other hand, a plus sign means that the system is electron stealing and your batteries are weak. When your cell voltage is a plus, you will not be able to generate the electrons you need to operate your electrical system or to create healthy new cells; this is *disease*. Keeping your pH in the normal, slightly alkaline range maintains your voltage in the normal range. This keeps your electrical system strong and healthy, therefore keeping you strong and healthy.

While cells normally operate at −20 to −25mV, making a new cell requires a much higher voltage: −50 mV. So unless your cell batteries are strong, and you are capable of producing and storing such a high voltage, you will be unable to make healthy new cells. To prevent repair deficits, to heal your body, and to stay young and healthy, you must be able to produce healthy new cells. In fact, the body must produce millions of healthy new cells every second of every day. If you are unable to create these cells, the result is repair deficits, degenerative disease, and aging.

When your pH is low (acidic) and your batteries are weak, your cells are unable to generate the energy they need to do their regular jobs, including the movement of nutrients into the cell and toxins out of the cell. This results in deficiency and toxicity—the two causes of all disease. Chronic disease is always defined by low voltage and low pH. For example, cancer patients typically have a voltage of +30 mV, which corresponds to a cellular pH of about 6.5 and a urine pH of 5.7, with terminal cancer patients often down to 4.5. Weak batteries and low pH are catastrophic to your health.

Measuring Your pH

Fortunately, pH is simple and inexpensive to measure. Anyone can do it with some pH paper, which you can buy at health food stores and at *www.beyondhealth.com*. If your pH is wrong, you can correct it. This puts you in charge of an extremely important determinant of health, contributing to your power to both prevent and cure almost any disease and to slow the aging process.

An indirect indicator of your body's cellular pH and voltage is the pH of your first morning urine, before you have had anything to eat or drink. This is an approximation of the alkaline reserves in your body and the strength of your batteries. Wet a small strip of the pH paper with urine and compare the color against the scale provided. Your test paper should be graduated from pH 5 to pH 8 with incremental readings. Always keep pH paper on hand, and have the whole family use it. It is estimated that at least half the U.S. adult population has a urine pH of 6.5 or lower, which helps explain our epidemic of chronic disease. Here is how to interpret your pH reading:

Below 6.5	Too acidic
6.5 to 7.5	Healthy range
Above 7.5	Too alkaline

When Your pH Is Too Low (Too Acidic)

Most chronically ill people have low pH. When your pH consistently measures below 6.5, you will begin to notice symptoms, such as fatigue, chronic pain, or frequent infections. As your pH continues to drop, the oxygen levels in your body will drop; you will get sicker and sicker, and you will be a prime candidate for cancer.

To control your pH, first pay attention to how your body is producing energy. If you are fatigued, hypoglycemic, or experience shortness of breath upon exertion, you may be producing energy through fermentation, which makes the body acidic. If your body has shifted to producing most of its energy through fermentation, you need to restore proper oxygen metabolism in your cells. Restore oxygen metabolism through detoxification, regular exercise, and supplementing with essential fatty acids, B vitamins, folic acid, CoQ10, magnesium, carnitine, and lipoic acid.

Avoid acid-forming foods such as sugar, grains, dairy, meat, and cola drinks. Eat an alkalizing diet with lots of fresh fruits and vegetables, preferably organic, and take alkalizing supplements. Alkalizing supplements include calcium, magnesium, potassium, and zinc in highly bioavailable forms. Keep a diary of the foods you eat and record your first-morning pH. This will allow you to monitor how different foods affect your pH. As you begin eating more foods that are alkaline and fewer acid-forming foods, you should see an improvement in your pH. To choose the right foods, see the acid/alkaline chart in Appendix B.

If diet and supplements are not able to control your pH, there are other factors to consider. Stress is one of them. Chronic stress creates acidity. Meditation techniques help to control this factor. Allergic reactions create acidity. Find out what foods you are allergic to and take care to avoid them. Avoiding just wheat and dairy can have a major positive impact for many people. Not only are these foods acid-forming to begin with, they are also highly allergenic. Chronic dehydration, many environmental toxins, most prescription drugs, and chronic infections all promote acidity. Chronic sinus infections or dental infections contribute to acidity and need to be addressed.

When Your pH Is Normal

If you have normalized your pH, congratulations! You are on your way to getting well and staying well. Monitor your pH regularly. First-morning pH should consistently run in the acceptable range. Occasional readings outside the acceptable range are okay, but consistent readings are not. If your pH falls below the normal range, follow the recommendations in the above section. Fortunately, you are in control of this critical factor, and you can use that control to choose health over disease.

Digestive Health

The digestive system is the most complex system in the body, and our health completely depends on it. Digestion also plays a huge role in immune function, with about 80 percent of immune activity located in the gut, and it directly impacts emotional and cognitive health. Unless you can properly digest and then assimilate nutrients from your food, there is no way you can be healthy. Symptoms of digestive malfunction include poor digestion, constipation, diarrhea, excess gas, belching, cramping, nausea, indigestion, acid reflux, bloating, abdominal pain, heartburn, bad breath, painful joints, chronic headaches, and vomiting. Many people think these digestive disorders are mere inconveniences. They are in fact symptoms of serious health problems and the warning signs of even bigger problems to come.

Unfortunately, most of us suffer from at least some degree of digestive malfunction. If you already have a health problem, to get well, you must place a high priority on improving digestive health. Our digestive problems have numerous causes, including the consumption of sugar, processed foods, prescription drugs, chlorinated water, GMO foods, and nonorganic meat and dairy products that are loaded with antibiotics. Regular use of antacids and thyroid deficiency both cause an insufficiency of hydrochloric acid in the stomach, which then results in maldigestion, poor nutrition, production of toxins, and numerous associated problems. But the largest single cause of digestive malfunction has been the irrational and irresponsible use of antibiotics by our obsolete and misguided medical establishment.

Few people, including most physicians, have an appreciation for the value of the microbes living in our digestive systems. The human body is home to trillions of microbes, living mostly in the gut. Your body has more microbes than human cells (they are smaller than human cells). These microbes act like another organ that performs tasks we need done but cannot do for ourselves. Gut bacteria do far more than help digest food; they have a major controlling effect on our physical and mental health. Our immune system depends on these microbes for many functions.

While all of us share similar microbes in our digestive systems, modern research shows that the makeup of this population is unique to each of us, unique as a fingerprint. Each of us is also biochemically unique, and our unique microbe population helps to support our unique biochemistry. Normally, these microbial communities remain stable over time. In fact, microbe populations even seem to run in families, similar to genes.

Problems arise when we damage the balance of these microbes, which can happen in a number of ways. Changing the pH of the gut diminishes levels of helpful bacteria. Prescription drugs such as NSAIDs and birth control pills also disrupt the balance. Drinking chlorinated water has a significant effect. Consuming nonorganic meat and dairy destroys beneficial bacteria due to the antibiotics they contain. However, the single largest problem is taking a prescription antibiotic; it is like dropping an atom bomb into this unique and vital community. Antibiotics indiscriminately kill everything in sight. Once this happens, your uniqueness is lost. As the microbe population reestablishes itself, you end up with a new set of players. Your original population that helped to keep you healthy and fight disease never returns to normal, and the new population opens the door to disease. This is why taking an antibiotic *even once* can damage your health for the remainder of your life.

For example, more and more studies are showing a relationship between antibiotic use and cancer. A study in a 2004 *Journal of the American Medical Association* determined that women who have taken antibiotics are at increased risk for developing breast cancer, and *as the number of prescriptions for antibiotics increased, the risk of breast cancer steadily climbed.* The researchers suggested that antibiotics kill off bacteria needed to metabolize and remove estrogen in the gut, which causes an excess of estrogen that stimulates cancer growth. Compared to women who took no antibiotics, those who had taken fewer than twenty-five antibiotic prescriptions had a 50 percent greater risk of breast cancer, while those who had taken more than twenty-five prescriptions had a 200 percent greater risk.

Antibiotic use is even causing infections. Widespread use of antibiotics creates antibiotic-resistant bacteria. These bacteria are now ravaging our hospitals and are moving out into the general population. They cause illnesses that are difficult, if not impossible, to treat with antibiotics.

The microbes in your gut even affect your weight. A normal, healthy microbe population digests more fiber and produces more short-chain fatty acids, which boosts calorie burning and causes less fat to accumulate. Obese people have fewer of these beneficial bacteria. A healthy diet filled with fresh vegetables increases the population of the microbes associated with leanness.

A properly functioning intestinal tract is one of your first lines of defense against disease, and declining levels of friendly intestinal bacteria precipitate the onset of chronic disease. A 2013 study in the *Proceedings of the National Academy of Sciences* showed that specific bacterial species within the gut are critical to protecting the airways against allergens and viral respiratory infection. By destroying the normal assortment of flora in the gut, antibiotics contribute to virtually every imaginable disease—from the common cold to autism, asthma, and psoriasis.

The disruption of intestinal flora, called *dysbiosis*, is a major contributor to our epidemic of chronic diseases such as accelerated aging, allergies, autoimmune syndromes, cancer, cardiovascular diseases, and neurodegenerative diseases. Dysbiosis disrupts your ability to digest food, assimilate nutrients, and eliminate waste products; it impairs the immune system, impairs the body's repair function, causes chronic inflammation, and accelerates the aging process. Dysbiosis can be measured with something called a CDSA (comprehensive digestive stool analysis) test.

Supplementing with fiber and beneficial bacteria has become a necessity to make up for our poor diets, stressful lifestyles, and use of prescription drugs. Avoid the use of antibiotics. There are a number of safe alternative treatments for infections, including vitamin C, olive leaf extract, and oil of oregano. Intravenous vitamin C, ozone, and ultraviolet light treatments can be used for serious infections. Supplemental digestive enzymes and hydrochloric acid are often necessary to address dysbiosis. However, all these must be of high quality, as most don't work very well. A good idea is to include raw, live-culture sauerkraut or kimchi in your diet.

Hormonal Balance

Hormones are part of the body's communication system. They are messenger molecules that provide instructions to help the body self-regulate. For example, when you eat sugar, insulin is released by the pancreas to instruct cells to take up sugar to restore proper blood sugar levels. However, insulin helps to manage many other things, including fat storage and the conversion of proteins to fat for storage. When you artificially increase insulin by eating sugar, you send out a lot of unintended messages. This upsets estrogen and testosterone levels in the body. In fact, eating sugar upsets your entire hormonal balance, sending a flood of incorrect messages throughout the body, throwing the body out of self-regulation. This reason is one of many that sugar is so danger-ous and deadly.

The body uses about fifty different hormones to help self-regulate. All of these are in a delicate balance with each other. Most people today suffer from hormonal imbalances, throwing their bodies out of self-regulation. Hormones act as genetic switches, activating certain genes and deactivating others. It is extremely important to your health that you normalize hormone function. The correct hormonal balance is antiaging, and the wrong balance speeds up the aging process. Hormonal balance is why getting the right amount of sleep is so important and why stress hormones can kill you. It is also why consuming meat and dairy products, and the hormones they contain, contributes to aging and disease. Our problems result from mineral deficiencies, improper pH of tissue fluids, poor diets, toxic exposures, prescription drugs, and exposure to hormonelike chemicals in our environment.

Particularly alarming is our ever-increasing exposure to hormonelike, endocrine-disrupting chemicals (EDCs). EDCs mimic hormones and give all the wrong signals to our genes. Increasingly, EDCs are turning up in scientific studies as causes of birth defects, infertility, diabetes, cancer, and even obesity. Even very low dose exposures to these chemicals can cause long-term health problems. Yet endocrine disrupters are everywhere, and other than taking bisphenol A out of baby bottles, the FDA has done almost nothing to protect us. These chemicals are present in almost all canned foods and beverages, cosmetics, sunscreens, pesticides, plastic water bottles, other plastics, food packaging, clothing, furniture, and the paper receipts one gets from stores, restaurants, and gas pumps. As much as possible, protect yourself from exposure to EDCs. *Do not drink from plastic bottles, do not consume canned foods and beverages, eat only organic meats, and do not store foods in plastic wraps.*

Thyroid Malfunction

Thyroid malfunction is epidemic today. This manifests as either too much or, in about 80 percent of cases, too little thyroid hormone. Low thyroid affects approximately 20 to 25 percent of the female population and about 10 percent of males. An additional 30 percent of persons over the age of thirty-five may also have subclinical or mild hypothyroidism.

Every cell in the body uses thyroid hormone to regulate numerous metabolic processes. Typical symptoms of malfunction include fatigue, sensitivity to cold, cold hands, hair loss, weight gain, dry skin, digestive problems, depression, and achy joints and muscles.

Like any disease, thyroid malfunction is the result of cells malfunctioning due to deficiency and toxicity. One of the most critical deficiencies is iodine. In 1999, global health experts announced that iodine deficiency continues to be a serious threat to global health; about 12 percent of Americans have been found iodine deficient. Selenium is another key thyroid nutrient, yet the majority of the U.S. population lives in areas having less than optimal selenium levels in their soils. Other key nutrients that support the thyroid include zinc, B vitamins, and vitamins C, D, and E. Omega-3 fats and amino acids are also essential, and coconut oil is helpful.

In addition to deficiency, toxicity also has a huge effect on thyroid function. This delicate system is easily disrupted by toxic chemicals from the environment. Chemicals such as phthalates, flame retardants, and bisphenol-A are known to disrupt thyroid function. Phthalates are found in many plastic products as well as fragrances and personal care products. Flame retardants are in furniture, carpets, upholstery, clothing, mattresses, electronics, and more. Bisphenol-A is present in plastic water bottles, food packaging, toys, paper receipts, dental sealants, and more.

Fluoride and perchlorate are both thyroid inhibitors and are found in tap water, which is one of many reasons that we need to filter tap water.

Pesticides also inhibit the thyroid, and they are found in tap water as well as in food.

Be aware that, even at very low levels, environmental chemicals can impact your thyroid function, and even small changes in thyroid function damage your health. This is just one more reason to reduce your exposure to environmental toxins.

Another source of thyroid malfunction is autoimmune disease, such as Graves' disease and Hashimoto's thyroiditis. Gluten and the artificial sweetener aspartame are thought to trigger autoimmune response in the thyroid.

In addition to paying attention to deficiency and toxicity, regular exercise is critical for optimal thyroid function.

Platelet Stickiness

Platelets are cell-like particles in the blood that form clots to prevent sudden blood loss in the case of injury. However, if blood clots form when they are not needed to stop bleeding, they can cause heart attacks and strokes, and even contribute to the cancer process. Platelets have sticky surfaces, allowing them to stick to each other and to other surfaces. Blood cells that are sticking together absorb less oxygen and deliver less oxygen. Even very small clumps of platelets can block smaller capillaries, causing less oxygen to be delivered to the cells that those capillaries serve. Less oxygen affects the body's ability to create energy and perform needed functions, and can lead to the formation of cancer cells.

As important as platelet stickiness is, few physicians appreciate its importance and do a platelet aggregation assay test. Most people can tell you what their cholesterol number is, which is not an important number, yet almost no one can tell you what their platelet aggregation number is, which is an important number. Platelet aggregation levels help to explain why some people with high risk factors—such as high blood pressure, high cholesterol, and blood vessels filled with plaque—never get a heart attack, while some people with none of those factors suffer massive heart attacks. People with the sticky platelets get the heart attacks and strokes. High platelet aggregation has even been associated with migraines and multiple sclerosis. Next time you see your doctor, be sure to get your platelet aggregation measured.

Small clots restrict blood flow into capillaries and deprive cells of needed oxygen. Less oxygen helps to switch cancer on, and the restricted flow also provides an opportunity for cancer cells that have broken off from a tumor to stop moving with the blood flow and start new tumor growth in other places in the body. Cancer deaths could be sharply reduced if these clots were eliminated. Maintaining good blood-flow speed helps to keep tissues well oxygenated. When people die of cancer, 90 percent of the time, they are succumbing to metastases, cancer cells that took root in other parts of the body after being shed by a primary tumor. Cancer cells that would normally travel through the capillaries are held up by the small clots and are able to attach themselves to the blood vessel wall and invade neighboring tissues, which helps to drive the cancer process. Fast-moving blood lessens this opportunity.

Platelet stickiness is caused by the same biologically inappropriate supermarket fats and oils that compromise the integrity of cell membranes, which is why platelet stickiness increases after consuming a typical American meal. Consuming essential fatty acids (EFAs) reduces platelet stickiness, provides good oxygen transfer, and increases blood speed, which reduces the ability for cancer cells to attach and invade new tissues. The EFAs in fish oil and flaxseed oil make platelets slippery so that they don't stick together. These oils have been shown in numerous studies to dramatically reduce the risk of clots. They also reduce inflammation.

Another source of clots is excess sodium. Excess sodium changes the electrical properties of cells, causing them to become less repellent and, therefore, more likely to stick together. Also contributing to stickiness are smoking, excess alcohol, and iron deficiency.

Sugar causes clots. Eating sugar and refined carbohydrates causes a rapid and dangerous increase in blood sugar. The body responds to this crisis by secreting insulin from the pancreas. Insulin promotes clotting. High insulin inhibits the breakdown of fibrin. Fibrin is the principal component of blood clots, and when it can't be broken down readily, clots can result. Because diabetics have high insulin, they have more blood clots and suffer more heart attacks and strokes. Eating a diet containing sugar, fruit juices, and refined grains increases insulin and promotes blood clotting. Anything that makes your blood insulin levels go up causes platelet stickiness, which is one more reason that sugar is a deadly poison.

Another problem with sugar is that when you increase the amount of sugar in the blood, the sugar reacts with proteins in the blood in a process called glycation. This has the effect of thickening your blood and making it flow less freely. Clearly, sugar should be eliminated from your diet, along with other "high-glycemic" foods such as grains, baked goods, sodas, and fruit juices.

Olive oil should play a prominent part in any healthy diet. Its anti-inflammatory and antioxidant effects result in a vascular environment in which platelets are less likely to clump together and form clots. Olive oil is also rich in inhibitors of platelet activating factor (PAF), which begins the clotting process by causing blood platelets to stick together. However, to get the benefits of olive oil, you have to get real olive oil instead of the usual adulterated oils that masquerade as "extra virgin olive oil" at the supermarket. (See Appendix A for high-quality olive oil.)

Supplementing with vitamin C, vitamin B6, essential fatty acids, and ginger substantially helps to prevent clots. For those on blood-thinning drugs, work with your doctor to wean yourself off the toxic drugs and substitute with antifibrin enzymes, such as nattokinase, to reduce the risk of clotting as well as cancer metastasis. Curcumin is especially good at reducing the high fibrinogen levels that promote clotting. Ginkgo biloba is a good blood-thinning herb. Like olive oil, it inhibits PAF, decreasing clotting and improving circulation. Ginkgo is also an anti-oxidant, and it reduces high cholesterol. Vitamin E also helps to prevent clotting; most of us are deficient in vitamin E. Magnesium slows clotting speed and stimulates fibrinolysis (the breakdown of fibrin and clots); most of us are deficient in magnesium. Garlic also reduces platelet stickiness and clotting.

Fat Storage

Most people look at being overweight as a cosmetic problem. To the contrary, overweight is a serious chronic disease caused by a malfunction in fat storage regulation. Fat storage is out of control in more than two out of three Americans because deficiency and toxicity have disrupted their ability to regulate and balance this body function.

Your body is programmed to regulate and balance appetite, fat storage, fat burning, and weight, along with body temperature, blood pressure, blood sugar, hormonal balance, and thousands of other factors. When fat storage regulation is disrupted by deficiency and toxicity, the resulting excess fat creates a cascade of consequences. It disrupts normal body chemistry, accelerates aging, and causes a wide variety of disabilities and health problems, including cancer. *Being overweight promotes platelet stickiness and blood clots. Fat cells in overweight people produce estrogen, disrupting hormonal balance and increasing the risk of blood clots and certain cancers. Fat cells also produce a flood of inflammatory chemicals, promoting systemic inflammation. Excess fat is a disaster.*

Numerous studies have proven that overweight people suffer from higher rates of cancer, heart disease, high blood pressure, diabetes, high cholesterol and triglycerides, breathing disorders, sleep disorders, arthritis, asthma, kidney stones, premature aging, and early death. Obese mothers are at least twice as likely to have children with debilitating birth defects. If you are overweight, your life expectancy is reduced.

Very simply, lean people live longer and have less disease, more energy, and a higher quality of life. This is why maintaining normal weight is so very important. A number of studies, including the Nurses' Health Study, a large ongoing health study that began in 1976, have shown that the leanest 20 percent live the longest, with mortality increasing progressively for each added pound. Perhaps even more important than living longer, lean people have higher-quality lives because they suffer less disability and dependence on others. Even if you are only ten pounds overweight, you are at risk for increased health problems, more disability, and shorter life.

Healthy people are not overweight, and overweight people are never truly healthy. Having excess weight is not just a cosmetic problem; it is a disease that makes you old and sick. In fact, predicting long-term health may be as simple as taking a waist measurement. Fat around the waist has been linked to higher mortality and the long list of diseases cited above. But the good news is even modest weight reduction can have significant health benefits, including lower triglycerides and cholesterol and better blood sugar balance. Some diabetics can even go off insulin.

In my book *Never Be Fat Again*, I identified overweight as a serious chronic disease caused by deficiency and toxicity. Recognizing overweight as a disease opens a world of possibilities, not only for weight management, but also for ending our epidemic of chronic illness. When you make yourself overweight, you throw your body out of balance. *Your* job is to help your body to do *its* job by keeping it balanced and properly self-repairing and self-regulating. When you interfere with the body's self-regulating systems by eating a poor diet, creating nutritional deficiencies, and exposing yourself to toxins, you *will* get sick—guaranteed.

Use the Six Pathways

The above maintenance items address major health issues and some very fundamental biochemistry. Controlling them is critical if you want to get well, stay well, and never be sick again. *This can be done by using the Six Pathways to health and disease.* By moving yourself toward health on each Pathway, you will automatically perform your required maintenance. This will allow you to become biologically younger, healthier, and filled with vitality. The Pathways offer a comprehensive program to empower you to create health and increase the length and quality of your life. If you are moving toward health on all six Pathways, you can't lose.

At the end of each Pathway chapter, you will find a list of the above maintenance items and a reminder of how choices you make can affect them for better or worse. This will provide you with a simple reference to help you control your maintenance and never get sick again.

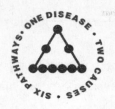

FIVE

Toxic Foods to Avoid

The well-nourished American is a myth.
Despite the high level of education and the abundance
of available food, many people make poor food choices
and are badly nourished. . . . The average human diet,
nutritionally unfit for rats, must be equally unsatisfactory
or even more so in meeting human needs.

—Carl Pfeiffer, M.D., Ph.D.,
Mental and Elemental Nutrients

The most basic weapons in the fight against
disease are the most ignored by modern medicine:
the numerous nutrients the cells of our bodies need.
If our body cells are ailing—as they must be in disease—
the chances are excellent that it is because they
are being inadequately provisioned.

—Roger J. Williams, Ph.D.,
Nutrition Against Disease

This first of two Nutrition Pathway chapters addresses what *not* to eat. While many modern foods fail to deliver the nutrition your body requires, certain foods are not only poor sources of nutrition, they are toxic and do you harm. By avoiding these toxic foods, you will go a long way toward improving your health. In fact, the improvement can be truly dramatic.

You are what you eat! There is no way of getting around this biological fact of life. Your body is made out of the building blocks you supply to it. If you eat junk, you will be made of junk. Good nutrition keeps you in good repair and working order. Yet, because we don't practice good nutrition, we have come to accept as normal the need for a knee or hip replacement or the likelihood that we may end up in a nursing home, unable to care for ourselves.

Today, more and more people complain of feeling sick and tired, while they continue to eat toxic, make-believe foods that do not and cannot support human health. Each of the trillions of cells in your body must be supplied with its daily needs or you cannot be healthy. Because we are not doing this, we are getting sick more often, getting old sooner, and becoming dependent on prescription drugs and replacement parts.

We need to turn this around. The simple solution is to change your eating habits. Eat better to live better. By choosing a better diet, you will boost your body's defenses, become stronger, and live longer. It is actually possible to live a disease-free life, never having as much as a cold. Try it; you will be sure to like it.

Deficiency is one of the two causes of all disease. Cells have a long grocery list of nutrients that you must deliver. Some nutrients, such as oxygen and water, are more urgent and must be delivered constantly or you will die within minutes or days. Most nutrients are less urgent, but must nonetheless be consistently delivered, or your cells will malfunction, and you will get sick. That's why eating a good diet is the single most important thing anyone can do to be healthy. *Yet the biggest impediment to improving health is that most people think they are already eating a good diet. The fact that only a small percentage of us actually eat a good diet helps to explain why chronic disease is rampant.*

Dr. Michael Colgan, author of *The New Nutrition*, had this to say: "Every year over 97% of your body is completely replaced, even the structure of the DNA in your genes, reconstructed entirely from the nutrients we eat. The quality of those nutrients determines the quality of your renewed cellular structure, the level at which it can function, and its resistance to disease."

To be healthy, each day, old worn-out cells must be replaced with new ones, and each new cell must perform all its intended functions. To build healthy new cells and have them carry out their many essential tasks, you need to supply the correct raw materials. To get those raw materials, you need to eat the right foods—foods whose calories are packed with the nutrients required to build and operate healthy cells. A diet consisting of processed foods does not and cannot supply what you need. If your diet includes foods such as ice cream, doughnuts, bread, pasta, potato chips, pizza, French fries, and coffee, you are making yourself sick. These so-called foods offer few nutrients and are loaded with toxins. To get what your body needs, each calorie you consume must be packed with nutrients and free of toxins.

Remember that a chronic shortage of even one nutrient will eventually make you sick, and most Americans are chronically short of at least several. You may be unaware that you are deficient, particularly at the early stages. However, when shortages are chronic, the body will no longer adequately repair and self-regulate. At some point you will become aware that all is not well, yet never stop to think that your poor diet is to blame. Then when you develop arthritis, cancer, diabetes, or some other chronic disease, your doctor will almost certainly blame your genes and your age, not your diet.

Building healthy cells starts in a mother's womb. If an embryo suffers from a shortage of building materials or the presence of toxins, a child with birth defects will be the result. During pregnancy, certain parts of the fetus are being constructed during specific weeks—such as the brain and nervous system, the circulatory system, and the digestive system. If essential raw materials are unavailable at that crucial time or toxins are present, any of these systems can be affected, perhaps manifesting as heart defects, digestive problems, lower IQ, attention deficit disorders, and so on. If any body system is not constructed properly in the first place, it will never work as well as it should. In extreme situations, the mother's body realizes that it is creating a defective product and rejects it. The construction process is shut down, and the fetus is aborted—an ever-increasing occurrence in our society. A 2010 study in *PLOS Genetics* concluded that a mother's nutrition in the days and weeks around the time of conception could have a lifetime effect on the way genes function in the child. Nutritional deficiencies in the fetus will affect its lifelong health.

A newborn baby's health is the product of the genetic material from both parents, plus the quality of available building materials (nutrients), minus the presence of toxins during gestation. People wrongly assume that genetics is the sole explanation for the health or disease of their children. Congenital defects (those present at birth) are not necessarily the result of genetics. For example, a 2001 *Lancet* reported a study regarding supplemental vitamins taken during pregnancy. Mothers who had taken both folic acid and iron supplements during pregnancy gave birth to children who were 60 percent less likely to develop the most common form of childhood leukemia. Eating right is especially important for expecting moms. Like any disease, leukemia doesn't "just happen." We create these diseases.

Trouble begins when your cell factories are supposed to be making some essential chemical but are not making enough of it because of a nutritional deficiency or toxicity. For example, if cells lack the raw materials to make sufficient antibodies for the immune system, we become more susceptible to infections. When cells lack the nutrients to make sufficient neurotransmitters, mental function suffers. (Neurotransmitters are chemicals generated by nerve cells that send information throughout the nervous system, allowing us to think, learn, and remember.) Hormones are another important part of the body's communications network. Hormones are chemicals that keep the body in regulation by traveling through the blood and lymph systems to bring messages to other parts of the body. When nutrient deficiency and toxicity prevent sufficient hormones from being produced or interfere with their operation, the body goes out of regulation. Today, hormone imbalance is epidemic.

Although each cell is a living entity unto itself, bodily systems can be regulated and controlled only when cells are able to communicate with each other. *Impairment of cellular communications is one of the most basic common denominators of disease, no matter how the disease happened or what it is called.* Cellular communication and feedback systems regulate everything from body temperature to immunity to movement. When these systems break down gradually, as they often do in disease, we may not notice until the condition is advanced. We are more familiar with sudden and severe breakdowns in bodily communication, such as spinal injuries that cause paralysis. We fail to recognize how subtle communication breakdowns precipitate chronic health problems.

As your body makes its hundreds of billions of new cells each day, it can make healthy cells or defective cells. Each time you order at a restaurant, each time you reach into your cabinet for a cooking oil, and each time you plan your day's meals, you are deciding whether you will build strong cells or weak ones. It is that simple, and the choice is yours to make. Are you going to maintain a strong body or cause it to become diseased and fall apart?

The Bad Four—What Not to Eat

Certain foods are so toxic that they damage the body faster than it can be repaired. This causes aging and disease. The easiest way to make your body fall apart is to eat a lot of what I call the Bad Four. The incidence of chronic disease has steadily increased along with the increased consumption of the Bad Four. The Standard American Diet (SAD) is loaded with the Bad Four, which is why the SAD does not support healthy life, even in laboratory rats. The Bad Four are sugar, wheat, processed oils, and dairy/excess animal protein. Let's have a look at these four deadly food choices.

Sugar

If you care about your health, get the sugar out of your life. Sugar either causes or contributes to every imaginable disease, from the common cold to cancer to Alzheimer's. It is a dangerous metabolic poison that makes you old and sick. Every time you consume sugar, you are doing damage to your body. It is difficult to think of a single food that is more dangerous, more destructive to human health than sugar. Dr. Linus Pauling, a chemist and twice Nobel laureate, once said, "Sugar is the most hazardous foodstuff in the American diet."

Sugar negatively affects every item on your Maintenance List, which is why getting it out of your life is so beneficial. Here is some of what sugar does:

- Damages energy production
- Causes inflammation
- Upsets normal pH
- Interferes with digestion
- Throws hormonal balance into chaos
- Causes platelet stickiness
- Causes overweight

Sugar is more damaging to health than alcohol or tobacco, yet children are allowed to purchase candy, ice cream, sodas, and other products containing this deadly toxin. Sugar has been found to be more addictive than heroin. Unlike other hazardous substances, sugar is unregulated—and even subsidized by the federal government with price supports. Shame on our elected officials! Eating refined sugar is a relatively new development in the history of the human diet, and the body is not designed to handle it. When forced to metabolize it, the body compensates to the best of its ability, but the results are catastrophic for your health. For example, high blood sugar causes a variety of brain malfunctions, and some researchers now refer to Alzheimer's as type 3 diabetes.

Even one teaspoon of sugar will damage your health, and most Americans eat and drink about twenty-two teaspoons of sugar every day—triple what they consumed just three decades ago. Teenage males consume about thirty-four teaspoons. It adds up quick. A glass of orange juice has six teaspoons of sugar. A serving of sweetened cereal has five teaspoons, and typical granola has six. Sodas are the largest single source of sugar in the American diet, yet sweetened yogurts can have more sugar than a can of soda. Most people are unaware of the various ways sugar sneaks into their diets, hiding in breads and cereals and processed foods. Oftentimes, it appears in disguise on food labels under names like sucrose, glucose, fructose, maltose, hydrolyzed starch, invert sugar, corn syrup, and honey. About 80 percent of processed foods contain added sugar.

A teaspoon or two of refined sugar is sufficient to disrupt normal body chemistry and throw you into biochemical chaos for a period of six to eight hours. Fat, carbohydrate, and protein metabolism; vitamin and mineral chemistry; immunity; digestion; hormonal balance; and homeostasis are all thrown into chaos every time you eat sugar. Eating sugar several times throughout the day, as most people do, keeps your body in biological chaos all day, every day. Chaos is disease! Because sugar is so fundamentally disruptive to our chemistry, it can promote or cause almost any disease. It even interferes with the predigestive action of saliva, causing digestive problems.

Refined sugar is absorbed quickly, rapidly elevating the sugar level in the blood. Elevated blood sugar creates a biochemical emergency, and the body responds by secreting insulin from the pancreas. One of insulin's normal functions is to regulate blood sugar by signaling cells to absorb sugar and either burn it for energy or store it as fat. However, when blood sugar increases rapidly, excess insulin is produced, and your blood insulin level remains abnormally high for hours thereafter, which is one of the most damaging things you can do to your body.

Excess insulin creates a cascade of negative effects, starting with reducing blood sugar too much, causing hypoglycemia. This causes the brain to secrete glutamate, and high glutamate levels cause anxiety, agitation, anger, depression, panic attacks, and an increase in suicide risk. The hypoglycemia and emotional response to glutamate can create cravings, which often result in even more sugar being consumed. Producing excess insulin puts stress on the pancreas and interferes with digestion. Insulin is a powerful stimulator of fat storage and inflammation, as well as cancer growth and metastasis. Some researchers believe that insulin may be the single largest cause of chronic disease. Dr. David Katz, director of the Prevention Research Center at Yale Medical School and author of *Nutrition in Clinical Practice*, had this to say: "Is insulin *the* master control of all disease? I don't know, but it's certainly a candidate for that role." People who live the healthiest and longest eat the least sugar and have the lowest insulin levels.

Eating sugar is worse than eating nothing! In *A History of Nutrition*, Elmer McCollum cited experiments in which animals fed water alone lived substantially longer than those fed sugar and water. The body requires certain nutrients to metabolize the sugar you eat, including B vitamins, calcium, magnesium, chromium, and zinc. Refined sugar does not contain these nutrients, so the body robs them from your reserves, which creates deficiencies and throws the body out of balance, creating disease. The purpose of food is to supply nutrients, but sugar robs you of nutrients.

Sugar is acid-forming in the body, throwing your normal pH out of balance. Sugar is so rapidly absorbed into the bloodstream and distributed to body cells that insufficient oxygen is available to effectively burn and metabolize the sugar. The result is incomplete burning and formation of a toxic acid called *pyruvic acid*. When eaten daily, sugar causes the body to become too acidic, and the body pulls precious minerals such as calcium and magnesium from the bones and teeth to neutralize the acid, which can lead to osteoporosis. Meanwhile, pyruvic acid accumulates in the brain and nervous system, causing neurological diseases such as Alzheimer's.

Sugar interferes with vitamin C metabolism and depresses immunity by 50 percent within two hours after eating it. Sugar and vitamin C have a similar chemical structure and compete with one another to enter cells. When a lot of sugar is present, it wins, creating an artificial shortage of vitamin C inside the cell. Infection-fighting white blood cells require fifty times as much vitamin C as do other cells. When they don't get it, you become susceptible to colds, flu, and all types of infections as well as cancer. Sugar not only helps to cause cancer, it drives cancer once you have it because sugar is fuel for the cancer cells; the more sugar you feed them, the faster they grow.

Another way sugar damages our health is through a process called *glycation*. Glycation happens when a sugar chemically bonds to proteins, fats, enzymes, and even the DNA in your cells to form advanced glycation end products (AGEs). AGEs form inside the body and increase dramatically whenever you increase the sugar content of the blood. Glycation fundamentally changes functional proteins so that they can no longer accomplish their mission in the body, and the damage is permanent. Glycation stiffens joints, hardens arteries, weakens heart muscles, and causes skin to wrinkle and lose its elasticity. *Glycation ages you, and it happens every time you eat the deadly metabolic poison we call sugar.*

It has been known for decades that diabetics, due to their high blood sugar, age faster than nondiabetics, suffering problems related to their eyes, brains, vascular systems, and kidneys. However, you don't have to be a diabetic for glycation to damage you. Eating even a teaspoon of sugar is sufficient to raise the sugar content of your blood and create a lot of AGEs. A breakfast of eggs and orange juice puts sugar and protein into the blood at the same time, forming AGEs. A protein meal followed by a sugary dessert creates AGEs. AGEs are absorbed into various body tissues, where they remain for long periods, initiating inflammation and causing oxidative damage to the body, increasing your risk of Alzheimer's, diabetes, heart disease, stroke, kidney failure, neurological deterioration, cataracts, retinal damage, and vision loss.

Immune cells try to get rid of AGEs. However, if you eat a lot of sugar and create too many AGEs, the immune system becomes overworked, making you more susceptible to infections and cancer. Glycation also damages enzymes. Disabled enzymes shut down critical functions inside cells, including energy production and DNA repair.

AGEs are produced internally, but you can eat them as well. Every time you eat foods that have been caramelized or meats that have been browned, you increase the amount of AGEs in your body. Any protein-containing meal that is prepared at high temperatures is loaded with AGEs. AGEs form in foods during the cooking process, particularly as foods brown. If you must cook food, cook at lower temperatures, as in steaming, poaching, stewing, and slow cooking. Avoid high-temperature cooking, as in barbecuing, broiling, frying, grilling, and roasting. Do not brown or blacken foods. Common foods that are high in AGEs include bacon, hot dogs, cured and smoked meats, baked beans, and toast. Most restaurant foods are loaded with AGEs, and most processed foods contain ready-made AGEs.

Any food that spikes your blood sugar causes glycation, including natural sweeteners like honey, maple syrup, agave nectar, brown rice syrup, and fruit juices—even those 100 percent pure or fresh-squeezed. Fresh whole fruit is okay in moderation. The fiber in whole fruit slows down sugar's entrance into the bloodstream, making whole fruit safer than juice.

Although all sugars contribute to disease and aging, the latest research shows fructose to be uniquely damaging to our health. Fructose, the sweetest of the three simple sugars found in nature, is the predominant sugar in most fruits. It is also a main ingredient in most refined sweeteners, such as table sugar, honey, agave nectar, maple syrup, high-fructose corn syrup, and crystalline fructose. Fructose is in almost every kind of processed food.

All of the fructose you eat is broken down in the liver, compared to only 20 percent of glucose (another common sugar). That's a lot of work for your liver! What's more, fructose metabolism creates a long list of waste products and toxins, including uric acid, which drives up blood pressure and can cause gout. Metabolized fructose turns into VLDL ("bad" cholesterol) and triglycerides, which get stored as fat. The fatty acids created during fructose metabolism accumulate as fat in your liver and skeletal muscle tissues, causing insulin resistance and nonalcoholic fatty liver disease. Insulin resistance progresses to metabolic syndrome and then to type 2 diabetes. And, as if all the fat you gain from eating fructose wasn't enough, fructose interferes with leptin, the hormone that suppresses appetite, causing you to overeat. In addition, fructose causes a net loss of energy from the body. Metabolizing fructose requires the conversion of fructose to fructose-1-phosphate. This reaction is energy intensive and it drains ATP from the cell, lowering energy levels throughout the body. Fructose appears to be favored by cancer cells, speeding up the growth and spread of cancer.

The upshot is that our modern diet is literally supercharged with fructose, and we are seeing the consequences in our skyrocketing rates of chronic and degenerative disease. If you want to stay biologically young, maintain a healthy weight, and radically reduce your risk of diabetes, heart disease, and cancer, then you must eliminate all refined sugars from your diet and keep your daily consumption of fructose to a minimum. Limit your consumption of fructose to 25 grams or less per day. An average orange has about 6 grams, a banana 7 grams, and an apple 10 grams.

It is worth taking a closer look at high fructose corn syrup (HFCS). HFCS is in just about all processed foods manufactured in the United

States, including breads, breakfast cereals, lunch meats, yogurts, soups, sodas, condiments, and desserts. It is used to improve the flavor of most packaged "make-believe" foods, and it is so cheap that the incentive to use it is enormous. As long as it remains legal (and, remarkably, subsidized by the federal government), there is no reason for the processed food manufacturers not to use it. However, there are excellent reasons for you not to eat it if you care about your health. On top of being a refined sugar, HFCS—which is made from genetically modified, chemically processed corn—comes with its own unique set of poisons. One such poison is glutaraldehyde, which is one of the chemicals used to turn GMO corn into cornstarch and then into HFCS. Glutaraldehyde is so dangerous that small quantities can burn holes in the human stomach.

Between one-third and one-half of all HFCS-containing products on the market have tested positive for mercury contamination. Two of the chemicals frequently used in HFCS production contain mercury. In some cases, the level of mercury was high enough that a woman eating the average amount of HFCS in the American diet could ingest more than five times the maximum recommended upper limit of mercury. Mercury causes Alzheimer's, cancer, and many other diseases. In the hunt for sources of mercury toxicity, here's a big source that hasn't even been on the radar. A simple solution is to *stop eating high fructose corn syrup*.

One of the easiest things you can do to quickly improve your health is to eliminate all soda and sweetened beverages from your life. Americans consume about 160 pounds of added sugar every year, and a third of that is from soft drinks. Eliminating them is possibly the single best thing you could do to reduce your sugar consumption. Then, since most processed foods also contain HFCS, avoiding as many processed foods as possible is your next step.

I say eliminate *all* soda, because even though HFCS is clearly something you want to avoid, it may not be as bad as artificial sweeteners found in diet sodas. Aspartame, used in most diet sodas, is known to be particularly toxic. One of the breakdown products of this molecule is formaldehyde. Formaldehyde accumulates in our cells, where it damages DNA and causes cancer. Drinking even one can of diet soda can cause DNA damage that leads to cancer, and your risk increases with each can consumed. It is now well established that aspartame, an excitotoxin, causes brain cancer, lymphomas, and leukemias in experimental animals. Aspartame can penetrate the blood-brain barrier and damage the brain and nervous system. Aspartame also increases your risk of strokes and heart attacks. The FDA—which once listed ninety-two side effects from consuming aspartame, including seizures, sexual dysfunction, and sudden cardiac death—has received more complaints about aspartame than any other substance.

Another common sweetener is Splenda. Splenda is an unnatural, man-made chemical that affects the body in numerous ways. The side effects of Splenda include skin rashes/flushing, paniclike agitation, dizziness and numbness, diarrhea, swelling, muscle aches, headaches, bladder issues, and severe gastrointestinal problems. Animal studies show that Splenda reduces the amount of good bacteria in the intestines by 50 percent, increases the pH level in the intestines, and contributes to increases in body weight. Artificial sweeteners are not an option!

If we look at the diets of primitive peoples around the world, we find that human beings have thrived on a wide variety of different diets without suffering from the diseases of civilization we see today. Eskimos did quite well on a diet of primarily blubber, as did the Bantu on a primarily vegetarian diet. However, one thing common to all of these traditional diets is the absence of sugar.

A very inconvenient truth is that sugar is highly addictive and destructive. However, knowing this is like pulling back the curtain on the great mystery of why so many in our society are sick, suffering, and dying prematurely. You do not have to be one of them. If you don't want to make yourself old and sick, avoid sugar.

Wheat

To be healthy, get wheat out of your life. Wheat is another so-called food that negatively affects every item on the Maintenance List. Most people are aware that white flour is not the most nutritious food they can eat. Surprisingly, even products labeled as "whole wheat" or "whole grain" often contain mostly white flour. To make white flour, the whole grain is stripped of over twenty essential nutrients, including 72 percent of its zinc and 85 percent of its vitamin B6. Almost comically, when a handful of these nutrients are added back, the flour is called "enriched," when it is really impoverished. White flour is inflammatory and enormously damaging to human health, disrupting vitamin, mineral, and hormonal balance. The average American consumes about 200 pounds of this deadly junk food every year.

White flour is mostly starch, and it quickly metabolizes into sugar, *causing all the same problems as sugar*. Like sugar, white flour causes an increase in blood sugar and insulin, producing a flood of pro-inflammatory chemicals and free radicals. In fact, wheat contains an unusual type of carbohydrate called amylopectin-A, which has been found to spike blood sugar even worse than table sugar. For that matter, wheat-based foods such as breads and cereals cause higher blood sugar spikes than many other carbohydrate foods.

While the problems with white flour are well known, most people are unaware that grains themselves are a problem, and that *wheat is the worst and most dangerous grain of all.* Until about 10,000 years ago, humans didn't eat grains. Now, just eight grains provide over half of all the calories and half of all the protein consumed on the planet. Importantly, the wheat we eat today differs significantly from what our ancestors ate. Wheat has been hybridized to achieve higher yield per acre and higher protein content, and hybridized wheat was introduced into commerce without anyone questioning its safety. But small changes in the structure of a protein molecule can spell the difference between a healthy nutrient and a toxin, and modern wheat proteins are having a toxic effect.

A big problem with wheat is a protein called *gluten*, which is found in all types of wheat and in barley and rye. Gluten is a gluey substance that provides elasticity and structure to dough, but it is highly allergenic and inflammatory and can affect digestion and assimilation of nutrients. Historically, gluten was not the problem it is today. Small occasional amounts were tolerated. But today's hybridized, high-protein wheat contains up to 90 percent more gluten than traditional wheat, and we are eating wheat multiple times per day. As a result, the number of people with gluten sensitivity has skyrocketed, causing massive problems. Celiac disease is the most extreme reaction to gluten. However, even if you are not allergic to gluten, it can damage your gut by causing the space between the cells of the intestinal wall to expand. This effect dramatically increases the permeability of the gut, causing a condition called *leaky gut*. Researchers have estimated that as much as half the population may now be metabolically reactive to gluten. Gluten reactivity manifests as a wide range of health problems, including chronic depression, chronic fatigue, common colds, eczema, fibromyalgia, irritable bowel syndrome, lupus, thyroid disease, and rheumatoid arthritis. Meanwhile, most people suffering from gluten sensitivity are completely unaware of the root cause of their symptoms.

No one should be eating wheat or other gluten-containing grains. Immune reactions to gluten produce free radicals and chronic inflammation. They also make the body more acidic, changing your pH balance. Choosing a diet that does not promote inflammation is essential for a long, disease-free life. *Eliminating gluten is a foolproof way of getting a powerful inflammation promoter out of your life.*

However, another problem may be even worse than gluten. Wheat and other grains contain a class of proteins called *lectins*. Hybridized wheat, with higher protein content, also contains higher levels of lectins than the wheat our ancestors ate. Research presented in a 2008 *FASEB Journal*, a 2000 *Gut*, a 1999 *Lancet*, a 1995 *Pediatric Allergy and Immunology*, a 1993 *British Journal of Nutrition*, and numerous other sources indicate that lectins may be the biggest problem with grain consumption. Lectins are powerful natural insecticides that plants use to protect themselves. Lectins attach to receptor sites on the cell membranes of bacteria and fungi and disrupt their function. This protects wheat and other grains from insects and infection. But humans have the same receptor sites! Consuming hybridized, high-lectin wheat is having a devastating effect on human health.

When we eat wheat, the lectins damage our gastrointestinal tract, creating holes in the gut tissue, causing a leaky gut. Undigested molecules, including gluten, are now free to enter into the bloodstream. The immune system sees these molecules as invaders and attacks them, creating inflammation and allergies. Increased intestinal permeability is now recognized as causing a wide variety of chronic inflammatory and autoimmune syndromes, including inflammatory bowel disease, celiac disease, multiple sclerosis, and eczema. In fact, lectins can do direct damage to the majority of tissues in the human body, which helps to explain why chronic inflammatory diseases are more common in wheat-consuming populations. Even at exceedingly small concentrations, lectins stimulate the production of pro-inflammatory chemicals such as interleukins 1, 6, and 8 in intestinal and immune cells. The inflammation created by lectins damages DNA and accelerates aging.

Lectins damage the thymus gland, which is essential to immunity, and they directly damage immune cells in the blood. They damage the thyroid gland. Lectins have the ability to pass through the blood-brain barrier and directly damage brain cells by attaching to, and thus damaging, the myelin sheath coating on nerves. Lectins also exhibit insulinlike properties, which can cause insulin resistance (diabetes) and weight gain. Lectins damage joints by binding strongly to their connective tissues. Lectins also stimulate platelet stickiness and blood clots, contributing to the risk of heart attack and stroke. Moreover, lectin blocks hormones that regulate food consumption, leading to eating more and becoming overweight.

Unfortunately, lectins are highly stable molecules. They survive cooking, sprouting, fermentation, and digestion. We are now consuming a lot of high-lectin wheat, and the lectins are accumulating in our tissues, putting a continuous toxic load on us. Whole wheat contains more lectins than white flour, and ironically may be an even bigger threat to your health.

In the last 130 years, grain consumption has sharply increased and so have our rates of chronic disease. Now grains represent about half of all the food consumed. All plants contain natural toxins to protect them from viruses, bacteria, fungi, and predators. Our genes are well adapted to handle the toxins in fruits and vegetables, but not so for the relatively recent addition of the special toxins in grains. Anthropological evidence indicates that when we started eating grains about 10,000 years ago, our health declined—infant mortality increased, life span shortened, infectious diseases increased, and bone disorders and dental decay appeared. One reason is that grains contain phytic acid, which prevents the absorption of calcium, copper, iron, magnesium, and zinc, causing mineral deficiencies. Eating grains also causes insulin to spike, prompting a cascade of harmful reactions in the body.

Grains do contain useful nutrients, but cooking is usually necessary to make grains edible, and cooking diminishes nutritional value. Baked goods that contain yeast present a special problem. Many studies have linked bread and other bakery products with cancer because of the carcinogenic mycotoxins that baked products contain. Mycotoxins are metabolic waste products of the yeast used to make bread. Another problem with baked goods is the formation of carcinogenic acrylamides in the browned portions of baked goods.

Most people think of wheat as a good food. However, sufficient evidence exists that wheat is instead a toxin and a major cause of disease. Anyone with a chronic illness should avoid all products containing wheat and other gluten-containing grains like barley and rye. Corn has also been hybridized and genetically modified to where it is highly toxic. Corn is rich in lectins that are known to damage gut tissue and reduce absorption of key nutrients. Certain lectins are capable of killing brain cells, and the lectins in corn can be especially toxic to people with brain diseases such as autism. High-fructose corn syrup is also neurotoxic.

In the interests of living a long, disease-free life, most people would do well to either eliminate or at least minimize the consumption of all grains—most especially wheat. The safest choices would be occasional servings of buckwheat, amaranth, and quinoa.

Processed Oils

Oils are essential building materials to construct healthy cells and to create numerous chemicals the body needs. The correct oils in the correct amounts create healthy cells and a healthy you. The wrong oils have a bad effect on your maintenance list: energy production, inflammation, platelet stickiness, hormonal balance, and fat storage. That's why you need to know this: *almost any oil you buy at the supermarket is the wrong oil.* Likewise, the oils in processed foods or served in most restaurants are also the wrong oils. When you put the wrong oils into your body, it's like putting the wrong oil into your car's engine—you are going to damage the engine. The wrong oils include canola, corn, cottonseed, peanut, safflower, soybean, and sunflower oils; all hydrogenated oils; and even most olive oils. Putting the wrong oils into your body affects all of your biochemistry, making it difficult for anything to work right—this is disease. *If you want to be healthy or recover from a chronic illness, you need an oil change.*

Cell membranes (the wall separating the interior of the cell from the rest of the world) are constructed with oils. But they must be exactly the right oils because these membranes perform many critical tasks, including regulation of what goes in and out of a cell—the delivery of essential nutrients and removal of metabolic wastes. These complex tasks can only be performed well if the membranes are constructed of the correct oils. An extremely critical function of cell membranes is the storage of electricity. Properly constructed cell membranes act as capacitors (electrical components that store electrical energy), which allow a cell that normally operates at −20 to −25 millivolts (mV) to build up and store the much higher −50 mV voltage required to construct a healthy new cell. If you want to keep your body in good repair, this fact is critical. If you are eating the wrong oils, you will not be able to store sufficient voltage to create new cells. If you are unable to replace old cells with new ones, you will eventually fall apart, become disabled, and need others to care for you. Nursing homes are filled with such people.

To keep ourselves in good repair, we build millions of new cells every second of every day. Unless the correct cellular building materials are available, your body makes your new cells out of what is available. Think of building a new house out of cardboard instead of high-quality plywood because the plywood is unavailable, but the cardboard is. Building a cell membrane with the wrong oils interferes with the transport of nutrients into cells and of toxic wastes out of cells, which causes deficiency and toxicity and results in cellular malfunction and disease. Almost all the processed foods we eat—salad dressings, baked goods, chips, breakfast cereals, fast foods, and restaurant foods—are made with biologically incorrect oils.

Humans need specific oils called essential fatty acids (EFAs). There are two categories of EFAs: omega-3 and omega-6. We need both types, and both are healthy, but these oils need to be consumed in the proper ratio to each other. Humans evolved on a diet that had a near equal 1:1 ratio of omega-6 and omega-3 fats, and these specific oils must be available when new cells are constructed. However, most Americans consume far too much omega-6 and far too little omega-3. The current ratio in our diet is about 20:1, and for some people it's as bad as 50:1. It's so bad that about 90 percent of the U.S. population is deficient in omega-3 fatty acids. A 1991 study in the *World Review of Nutrition and Dietetics* showed that 20 percent of us have so little omega-3 in our blood that standard tests cannot measure it. Biologically speaking, this is a disaster, not only for adults, but also for the unborn. A mother whose diet is deficient in omega-3 fats produces babies with impaired immunity and increased risk of developing allergies, as well as impaired brain development and cardiovascular health.

Omega-3 oils have a measurable effect on brain performance. A 2011 study in *Neurology* confirmed that people with diets high in omega-3 fatty acids and in vitamins C, D, E, and B had higher scores on think-ing tests and were less likely to have the brain shrinkage associated with Alzheimer's disease than people with diets high in trans-fats. A 2012 study in *PLOS ONE* found that blood levels of omega-3 DHA predicted how well schoolchildren were able to concentrate and learn. Those with the lowest omega-3 levels had the poorest reading and memory skills and the most behavioral problems.

The imbalance of omega-6 and omega-3 oils in our diet causes chronic inflammation, and chronic inflammation causes chronic dis-ease. Both classes of EFAs produce body chemicals called *prostaglandins*. Inflammatory prostaglandins are produced from omega-6 fatty acids; they suppress the immune system and increase inflammation, heart dis-ease, cancer, and aging. Excess omega-6s dramatically lower the amount of vitamin E in the body, which increases free-radical damage to DNA and tissues, promoting the growth and metastasis of tumors. In addi-tion, fatty acid imbalance causes the clumping of red blood cells, which slows down blood flow, restricts blood flow to the smaller capillaries, and results in poor oxygen delivery to cells. When sufficient omega-3 oils are present, anti-inflammatory prostaglandins are produced, and these offset and balance those prostaglandins from the omega-6s. Anti-inflammatory prostaglandins from omega-3s suppress inflammation, tumor development, blood pressure, water retention, blood platelet stickiness, and cholesterol levels.

While the primary reason for the enormous imbalance of 6s and 3s in the American diet is the excessive consumption of the supermarket oils, a secondary reason is the decrease in the consumption of real fish, meat, and eggs. For example, most of the salmon and many of the other fish available today have been farmed in artificial environments. Farmed fish are fed grain, as opposed to the normal diet they would consume in their native oceans and rivers. As a result, they contain the wrong fatty-acid ratios because grains are high in omega-6s. The same holds true for beef and chicken, which are fed grains that change their fatty-acid ratios. Consider that a real egg, from a hen eating a natural diet, contains about 300 milligrams (mg) of the omega-3 fatty acid DHA (docosahexaenoic acid). Standard, grain-fed, supermarket eggs average only 18 mg of DHA, and they are high in omega-6s.

These omega-3-deficient, industrially produced foods are damaging our health. To compensate, we need to increase intake of omega-3 fatty acids. Flaxseed oil is one of nature's richest sources of EFAs. Flaxseeds, freshly ground in a small coffee grinder, make an excellent addition to fresh salads and smoothies. Other rich sources include wild-caught fish, green leafy vegetables, nuts, seeds, and EFA supplements.

Although cattle graze on grass for most of their lives, nearly all cattle are shipped to feedlots prior to slaughter to fatten them up on grain. If you eat this grain-fed beef, as most Americans do, you worsen your omega-6 to omega-3 fatty acid ratio. Natural beef (grass fed and grass finished) is rich in omega-3s, but grain-fed beef is rich in omega-6s. If you choose to eat beef, eat grass-fed/grass-finished, organic beef. Just eating organic meats is not good enough. That just means the animals were fed organic grains. The meat contains fewer pesticides but still has the wrong fatty acid ratio—grass-fed/grass-finished is what you want.

Another major problem with supermarket fats and oils is that commercial processing subjects them to heat, chemicals, and oxidation, significantly changing their molecular structure and making them toxic to the body. Most supermarket oils undergo a bleaching and deodorizing process to make them crystal clear and extend shelf life. This process usually takes place at high temperatures, at which massive trans-fat formation occurs and powerful toxins called *lipid peroxides* are formed.

There is no safe level of lipid peroxides or trans-fats. Also, because processed oils are stripped of their natural antioxidants, manufacturers add preservatives, which are toxic. Yet another problem is that about 40 percent of these oils, especially soy and corn oil, contain solvent residues from their manufacture, contributing to our toxic overload.

The fats we call *hydrogenated oils* are uniquely dangerous, and they are found in everything from baked goods to breakfast cereals to peanut butter. These liquid vegetable oils have been chemically altered to make them solid at room temperature. Such man-made fats contain unnatural molecules, including trans-fats that are toxic to your body. Some products are now being labeled as "trans-fat free," but this claim can be deceptive. Trans-fats have to be disclosed on the label only if the food contains more than 0.5 grams per serving. Even that amount is toxic, but to avoid listing trans-fats, or to claim "trans-fat free," on their labels, food manufacturers simply adjust the serving size until the trans-fat content falls under 0.5 grams per serving. Thus, modern food labels often have serving sizes that are much smaller than the amount you would normally consume. Be sure to read food labels carefully. Never eat anything containing any hydrogenated oils, which are sometimes listed as "margarine" or "vegetable shortening." A much better choice is coconut oil, which is a clean source of needed saturated fat and resists oxidation and degradation at higher temperatures.

Cells must create energy by combining a fuel (usually fats, sometimes carbohydrates) with oxygen. Enzymes play a crucial role in this process, and they are designed to fit and interact with very specific molecules. The problem with overprocessed supermarket oils is that processing changes the shape of the molecules, and the misshaped molecules do not fit the appropriate enzymes, so they cannot be processed into energy. You are supplying the wrong fuel!

Avoid supermarket oils, all hydrogenated oils, and all food products containing these oils. Avoid grain-fed animals, eggs, and fish; they are too rich in omega-6s. Instead, fill your grocery cart with fresh organic vegetables, fruits, raw nuts, wild-caught fish, and organic grass-fed meats. Choose olive, coconut, flaxseed, and fish oils, but these must be minimally processed, high-quality oils, and most brands do not measure up. Unfortunately, most olive oil is adulterated with toxic oils. Without the correct oils in your diet, aging is accelerated and you will get sick. *If you want to prevent or reverse chronic disease, you need an oil change.* (See Appendix A for acceptable oils.)

Dairy/Excess Animal Protein

Most of us have been brought up to think that milk is a good and necessary food. *Wrong!* We have been terribly misled into consuming milk and dairy products and far too much animal protein. Americans are among the world's highest consumers of milk products, and we consume about ten times too much animal protein.

Consuming milk is both unnatural and unhealthy. Nowhere in nature does one species drink the milk of another or drink milk after weaning. Only humans do these unnatural things, and we suffer the consequences with heart disease, osteoporosis, diabetes, infections, arthritis, allergies, and cancer. Most Americans have been brainwashed when it comes to dairy products. I certainly was. I grew up believing that milk, cheese, and yogurt were vital parts of a healthy diet. The first time someone suggested to me that dairy products were not healthy, I thought he was crazy.

When I tell people not to drink milk, they often ask, "Where will I get my calcium?" Seventy percent of the world's people do not drink milk. Where do they get their calcium? They get it from plant foods. Green vegetables, such as kale, broccoli, and collard greens, are loaded with calcium.

Milk and dairy products are not part of a healthy diet. Even back when most of us were farmers, traditional milk from one's own cow was not a healthy food choice, but it wasn't a deadly poison either. Modern milk, on the other hand, is a highly processed and allergenic make-believe food that is a threat to anyone's health.

Commercially produced milk is a toxic soup loaded with fifty-nine biologically active hormones, dozens of allergens, up to fifty-two powerful antibiotics, pesticides, herbicides, PCBs, dioxins (up to 200 times the safe levels), blood, pus, feces, solvents, viruses, excessive bacteria, and even radioactive compounds. Of those fifty-nine hormones contained in milk, one is the powerful growth hormone IGF-1 (insulinlike growth factor 1). IGF-1 is like rocket fuel for cancer. It instructs cells to grow. Instructing cells to grow may be fine for the calf, for which the milk is intended, but in adults, it promotes cancer. IGF-1 is known to be a factor in the rapid growth and proliferation of breast, colon, and prostate cancers, and most likely plays a role in all cancers. Men who consume two or more servings of milk per day have a 60 percent increased risk of prostate cancer. Ice cream is far worse. IGF-1 gets concentrated in the cream, and one serving of ice cream gives you twelve times as much IGF-1 as you would get in one serving of milk. Most men suffering from chronic prostatitis improve their condition by removing dairy from their diet. Another cancer promoter in milk is casein, the predominant protein in cow's milk. Casein promotes cancer at every stage in the cancer process. No one should be drinking milk or consuming products containing milk.

Virtually all milk is pasteurized and homogenized. This processing substantially changes the chemical and physical properties of the milk and, for many reasons, makes it less nutritious, more toxic, and more carcinogenic. Pasteurized milk is an acidic food. Most Americans are eating too many acidic foods already, and milk throws your pH balance further out of whack. In *Fit for Life: A New Beginning*, author and nutritionist Harvey Diamond states:

> *It is a well-established fact that the high protein content of meat and dairy products turns the blood acidic, which draws calcium out of the bones. This causes the body to lose or excrete more calcium than it takes in. The deficit must be made up from the body's calcium reserve, which is primarily the bones.*

Millions of us have paid a very high price for the misguided advice put out by the dairy industry. Advertising by the Milk Advisory Board and articles presented as news driven by the same interests tell us to drink milk to ensure proper calcium intake. Calcium is indeed needed, but drinking milk causes net calcium losses and osteoporosis. Yet people with osteoporosis are instructed to consume more milk! Vitamin D is critical for calcium metabolism, which is why most milk is "fortified" with vitamin D. However, a study in a 2001 *American Journal of Clinical Nutrition* found that people who consume the most milk actually have the lowest vitamin D levels. Industrial milk is not a good source of either calcium or vitamin D. Americans are among the biggest milk consumers in the world, and like other countries that have high consumption of dairy products, we pay a price with the world's highest rates of osteoporosis, diabetes, heart attack, allergy, and cancer.

Paul Nison, author of *The Raw Life*, stated, "Dairy is the cause of most disease in the world today." When a prominent Washington, D.C., pediatrician was asked in an interview what single change to the American diet could provide the greatest health benefits, Dr. Russell Bunai replied, "The elimination of milk products."

Excess Animal Protein Makes You Old and Sick

Protein is an essential nutrient, required to construct hormones, enzymes, and other indispensible molecules, as well as structural tissue. Without protein, life cannot be sustained. However, animal protein, in excess of the amount needed for growth, promotes aging and disease. Unlike plant protein, the animal protein in milk and meat metabolizes to strong acids—disrupting your acid/alkaline balance, lowering the pH of your cells, robbing your teeth and bones of minerals, and making your cell batteries weaker.

The Recommended Daily Intake (RDI) for total protein is 50 to 60 grams per day. Many Americans get twice this amount. Our average consumption of animal protein alone is about 70 grams per day—more than the RDI for total protein. By contrast, most rural Chinese, who are far healthier than we are, average 7 grams of animal protein per day (about the amount contained in one egg). Averaging 7 grams or less per day of animal protein is a worthy goal—approximately one egg or a piece of fish or meat the size of the palm of your hand. The remainder of the RDI should be plant protein from vegetables, nuts, seeds, sprouts, legumes, and avocados.

Excess animal protein promotes kidney, eye, and brain diseases; auto-immune disorders; obesity; heart disease; diabetes; osteoporosis; and cancer. A 2014 study in *Cell Metabolism* found that people who ate a diet rich in animal proteins were more than four times as likely to die of cancer as those who ate a low-protein diet. In addition, those who consumed diets high in animal proteins were several times more likely to die of diabetes, as well as 74 percent more likely to die prematurely from any cause. A high-animal-protein diet disrupts hormonal balance by increasing the ratio of estrogens in the body, which stimulates cancer. People who are on high-protein diets to lose weight need to be aware of this danger. Animal protein is also rich in a fat called arachidonic acid, which studies have linked to promoting tumor growth and metastasis.

Animal protein can be consumed safely and beneficially in small quantities. However, the source is important. A study by the Harvard School of Public Health concluded that a daily meal of hot dogs, bacon, or hamburgers raises the risk of dying from heart disease or cancer by as much as 21 percent. If you choose to eat meat, make sure it's unprocessed and organic. The fish you eat should not be farmed, and the eggs should be organic as well. A good rule is to use animal protein as a condiment, not as a main course. You do not need to consume animal protein at every meal or even every day. Most of your protein should come from plant-based foods. People have been so conditioned to think of meat and dairy as their sources of protein that they don't even think about the protein in plant foods. Who would guess that, calorie for calorie, spinach has as much protein as beef?

Excess animal protein is an important factor in causing chronic disease, including kidney and eye disorders, obesity, Alzheimer's, osteoporosis, diabetes, heart disease, and cancer. Plant protein does not have a cancer-promoting effect, and large amounts can be safely consumed.

Here are some ways to cut down on animal protein:

- Introduce more primarily vegetarian meals.
- Build meals around fresh raw salads as the main course. You can add a small amount of high-quality animal protein or protein-rich sprouts to your main-course salad.
- Avocados contain protein and good essential fats; they can be used to replace meat in meals.
- Nuts and seeds (raw and soaked/sprouted) are a good source of protein and healthy fat.
- Lentils can be easily adapted to replace ground beef in Mexican recipes, shepherd's pies, meatballs, and stuffed peppers.

If you do eat meat, make sure it is not grilled, charred, or blackened in any way. When fat drips into an open flame, dangerous carcinogens called *polycyclic aromatic hydrocarbons* are formed. All proteins cooked at high temperatures contain several chemicals proven to cause cancer in laboratory animals. Barbecuing is the worst way to prepare meat because of both the open flame and higher temperatures. When I cook meat, I slow cook it at a low temperature using a crockpot.

You can improve health and reverse aging by lowering the amount of animal protein in your diet. At least 90 percent of your protein should be derived from plant foods such as vegetables, gluten-free whole grains, legumes, lentils, seeds, nuts, and sprouts. Fish and seafood are healthy forms of animal protein. Unfortunately, seafood is becoming increasingly toxic and dangerous to consume. An occasional small portion of fresh fish would be okay, but farmed or canned fish is not a good option. Farmed fish contain a lot of toxins and the wrong fatty acid ratios. Canning depletes nutrients and introduces toxins.

Other Poor Choices

Beyond the Bad Four, other poor dietary choices include excessive amounts of salt, food additives, and genetically modified foods. To be healthy, these too must be avoided.

Excess Salt

Salt is sodium chloride, and eating too much salt results in excess sodium in your body. Sodium is an essential nutrient, and we need it to help our nerves function properly, to aid nutrient absorption, and to maintain the right balance of water and minerals in our bodies. But sodium works in tandem with potassium, and things go wrong when we upset the normal ratio of the two. Mother Nature tells us the balance of sodium and potassium we need. Human milk contains three times as much potassium as sodium, yet we get it wrong and average four times as much sodium as potassium.

The human body requires only about 220 mg of sodium per day. One teaspoon of refined salt contains 2,300 mg of sodium—about ten times what we need. The USDA *Dietary Guidelines for Americans 2010* recommends consuming less than 2,300 mg and acknowledges that older people, African Americans, and people with hypertension, diabetes, or kidney disease should limit their intake to 1,500 mg per day. Only about 5 percent of us are actually doing that.

Upsetting your sodium/potassium balance has serious biological consequences.

Excess sodium in the diet is a disaster for your electrical system. Salt has an acidic effect on the body, lowering pH, altering the acid/alkaline balance, and forcing more sodium into cells. The result is weakened cell batteries, a damaged electrical system for your body, and, among other problems, heart palpitations.

Natural foods that are rich in potassium and low in sodium are what we were designed to eat. Unfortunately, we have changed to a sodium-rich diet of processed foods, and it is making us sick. Even eating at a "healthy" salad-bar restaurant can be a health hazard. Consider this: If you have a bowl of split-pea soup, you consume 1,430 mg of sodium. A serving of a typical "healthy" nonfat Italian salad dressing adds another 1,350 mg. Two "healthy" low-fat muffins add another 1,400 mg. A serving of mushroom marinara sauce on your hot pasta adds another 318 mg. Choosing a couple of the salad offerings adds another 400 mg, and chocolate pudding for dessert adds another 177 mg. This adds up to a whopping 5,075 mg of sodium—at just one meal—more than twice the USDA guideline.

Some of the biggest sources of sodium are products made from grains, such as bread, pasta, and pizza crust. Tomato sauce and cheese add even more sodium. One slice of whole-wheat bread typically contains about 100 mg of sodium. There are 200 mg in one cup of cornflakes, and 709 mg in two ounces of turkey-breast lunch meat. Still more can be found in processed vegetables, including vegetable-based soups and sauces and canned vegetables, not to mention potato products such as chips and fries. There are 390 mg of sodium in a half-cup serving of canned peas and 780 mg in one cup of canned vegetable beef soup. One cup of low-fat milk contains 107 mg of sodium, and one ounce of cheddar cheese contains 180 mg.

When your sodium intake is too high, your bones get weak. For every 2,000 mg of sodium you eat, you will lose about 25 mg of calcium in your urine. Unless you replace the lost calcium—and most people don't eat enough bioavailable calcium to do that—then eating an average of 5,000 mg of sodium per day could result in calcium losses as high as 2.5 percent of your skeleton annually. At that rate, you will lose 25 percent of your bone structure in only ten years. Since bone loss is progressive, older people tend to have weak bones, and today even young people suffer from weak bones. Osteoporosis is just one more "disease of aging" that we ourselves create and can easily prevent.

Excess sodium also increases the risk of high blood pressure, which is a major cause of heart disease and stroke. In fact, people who consume more than 4,000 mg of sodium per day double their risk of stroke compared to those consuming less than 1,500 mg. Other ramifications of excess sodium include chronic fatigue, neurological disorders, cancer, weight gain, impaired immune function, platelet stickiness, and premature aging. Research reported in a 2013 *Nature* concluded that excess salt triggers an abnormal immune response, which is capable of causing autoimmune diseases such as multiple sclerosis, psoriasis, and rheumatoid arthritis.

Fast foods are loaded with salt. It takes a lot of awareness to eat a low-salt diet, but you can do it. In restaurants, soups often contain a lot of salt: Avoid them. Many restaurants use too much salt: Request less. Read labels carefully. To increase potassium, eat more fresh fruits, vegetables, nuts, and seeds. Foods that are high in potassium include bananas, oranges, avocados, tomatoes, broccoli, lima beans, melons, cucumber, papayas, mangos, kiwi, and spinach. These same foods contain many other nutrients that our bodies need to stay healthy and biologically young.

Food Additives—A Toxic Mix

In *Diet for a Poisoned Planet*, author David Steinman describes an experiment in which four sets of rats were fed different diets. The first set ate natural foods and drank clean water. Throughout the three-month experiment, these rats remained alert, calm, and social. The second set was fed the same food as the first, with the addition of hot dogs. These rats became violent and fought each other aggressively. The third set ate sugarcoated breakfast cereal and drank fruit punch. These rats became nervous, hyperactive, and aimless. The fourth set was fed only sugar doughnuts and cola. These rats had trouble sleeping, became extremely fearful, and were unable to function as a social unit. The poor nutrition of these foods, plus the effects of the toxic colors, flavors, preservatives, and other additives they contained, had a profound effect on the behavior of these animals. Why, then, are we surprised that our children are struggling with hyperactive, antisocial, and even violent behaviors? Why, then, when children commit violent acts, we jump to blame the gun or whatever weapon they used but never question their diets or the mind-altering prescription drugs they may be taking?

Avoiding toxic food additives is simple. Eliminate processed foods from your diet.

Glutamates

Glutamates are chemicals used in processed foods, fast foods, and restaurants to enhance the flavor of the food. They are among a class of compounds known to act as excitotoxins, exciting nerves to stimulate the sensation of flavor. The best-known form of glutamate is monosodium glutamate (MSG). Glutamates damage the brain and nervous system, causing problems such as migraines, seizures, learning disorders, Parkinson's, and Alzheimer's. Glutamates also cause diabetes, obesity, overweight, and heart attacks. Glutamates produce enormous amounts of free radicals in the body, resulting in inflammation. *Regular consumption of glutamate-containing foods damages your brain and your health.*

Most of us are exposed to glutamates daily because they are in about 80 percent of all processed foods. Glutamates are cleverly disguised on food labels with words such as "natural flavors," "spices," "hydrolyzed vegetable protein," "vegetable protein," "caseinate," "textured protein," "soy protein extract," "glutamic acid," and others. A restaurant menu or label that says "No MSG" may still be serving you food loaded with glutamates. Even baby formula can contain glutamate in the form of caseinate. When you start to look for it, you may be shocked at how often you will find glutamates. They are everywhere. Commercial pizza and most fast foods are known to have a lot.

GMO Foods—An Unfolding Disaster

Foods made with genetically modified organisms (GMOs) have been prohibited in countries around the world for a good reason: they are dangerous. Yet Americans are consuming them by the ton in the form of corn, soy, canola oil, cottonseed oil, sugar from sugar beets, and papayas grown in Hawaii. These find their way into all kinds of processed foods, including popcorn, soy sauce, tofu, frozen pizza, frozen dinners, breakfast cereals, baby formula, canned soups, cookies, and ice cream. Almost all processed foods at the supermarket contain at least some GMO components, unless they are 100 percent USDA Organic.

GMO foods are a threat to human health and to all life on the planet. Unlike natural plant breeding, genetic engineering happens in a lab, where cells undergo a gene insertion process that couldn't happen in nature. It can change the nutritional content of food, make the food more allergenic, and even create unique toxins, and that's just the tip of the iceberg. GMO crops appear to be an unfolding nightmare.

Every generation of GMO crops interacts with more organisms, creating more opportunities for unwanted side effects for every living thing on the planet. Yet this damage may take years to manifest and is difficult to trace back to the GMO food. Worse, it is not reversible. Recent studies have found accidentally inserted viral fragments in commercial GMO crops that have unknown and perhaps dire potential consequences for both agriculture and human health.

Animal studies from around the world have shown GMO crops to be extremely dangerous, causing damage to the liver, heart, lungs, kidneys, adrenal glands, intestines, spleen, and pancreas. They shorten life and promote massive tumors. GMO soy and corn fed to test animals cause stomach inflammation, thinning of intestinal walls, hemorrhagic bowel disease, and higher rates of miscarriage. The introduction of foreign genes changes the entire nature of plant biology, turning food into a disguised poison that can potentially contaminate the genetic code of other plants and animals, including us.

Genetically modified plants can be designed to produce internal pesticides that we then eat. Such is the case with Monsanto's GMO corn. The corn's DNA is equipped with a gene from soil bacteria called *Bt* (*Bacillus thuringiensis*) that produces the pesticide Bt-toxin. Monsanto claims the toxin is harmless to humans because it's destroyed during digestion. It isn't. Bt-toxin has shown up in the blood of pregnant women and their babies.

Another problem with GMO foods is they contain glyphosate residues. Glyphosate is the active ingredient in Monsanto's herbicide Roundup—the most common weed killer in the United States. If you are consuming foods containing wheat, sugar, corn, or soy, unless they are organic, they will contain glyphosate residues. Glyphosate is a hormone disrupter and has been clearly linked to infertility and miscarriage in cattle, horses, pigs, sheep, and poultry that are raised on GMO feed. Glyphosate has been linked to hormone-dependent cancers, even at extremely low levels. A 2013 study in *Entropy* concluded that glyphosate may be "the most important factor in the development of multiple chronic diseases and conditions that have become prevalent in Westernized societies." The study further concluded that glyphosate may "enhance the damaging effects of other food-borne chemical residues and toxins in the environment to disrupt normal body functions [including gut bacteria] and induce disease."

Glyphosate is a strong chelator, meaning it immobilizes critical micronutrients, making them unavailable to a plant that has been sprayed. As a result, the nutritional content of GMO plants is profoundly compromised, and the health of people who consume the plant is compromised as well. Essential micronutrients such as iron, manganese, and zinc can be reduced by as much as 80 to 90 percent in GMO plants.

Glyphosate can accumulate and persist in the soil for years, where it kills off beneficial microbes and stimulates disease-causing pathogens. It is even causing the emergence of superweeds that the glyphosate can't kill. When applied to crops, glyphosate becomes systemic throughout the plant, so it cannot be washed off. Once you eat this crop, the glyphosate ends up in your gut, where it can decimate your beneficial bacteria. Just as glyphosate kills soil bacteria that are crucial for plant health and nutrient uptake, it also kills beneficial bacteria in your gut, which can wreak havoc with your health, as 80 percent of your immune system resides in your gut and is dependent on a healthy ratio of good and bad bacteria. Glyphosate damages digestive health—a seriously overlooked mechanism by which it damages human health overall.

Since the U.S. Food and Drug Administration doesn't require GMO foods to be labeled or tested for safety, the simplest way to avoid them is to buy whole, certified organic foods. By law, foods that are certified organic must never intentionally use GM organisms and must be produced without artificial pesticides and fertilizers. Certified organic animals must be reared without the routine use of antibiotics, growth promoters, or other drugs. Unfortunately, even organic crops are now being unintentionally contaminated with GMOs, which is why organic soy and corn are not necessarily safe to eat. As a practical matter, all U.S.–produced corn and soy should no longer be considered foods fit for human consumption. Drastically reduce your exposure to GMO foods.

Genetic engineering is mad science, and it's absolutely unnecessary. Safe organic farming methods allow us to grow sufficient food without poisoning our environment and our bodies.

Alcohol

Alcohol is not a food. It is a toxin. Alcohol is extremely toxic to virtually every organ system; it poisons and impairs the function of the brain, heart, liver, kidneys, lungs, gut, and pancreas. It depresses the central nervous system and impairs judgment and functioning, causing accidents and injuries. A 2013 study in the *American Journal of Public Health* found that alcohol is to blame for one in every thirty cancer deaths in the United States. The connection was especially powerful with breast cancer, where 15 percent of those deaths are alcohol related, and 30 percent of these alcohol-related deaths were linked to drinking 1.5 or fewer drinks per day.

Dr. Judith Hall, a geneticist at the University of Washington, estimates that alcohol-related birth defects may be as high as one or two per 100 births. As few as two drinks per day has been associated with low birth weights and a higher rate of stillbirths. Even social drinking can be a problem, producing defects of varying severity such as hyperactivity and learning problems. In fact, there is no safe level of alcohol consumption during pregnancy. Since many women are not aware of their pregnancy for two months or more, and since the first trimester is a particularly critical time, women wishing to have children must be especially careful. Would-be fathers must also not drink alcohol. Alcohol can damage the quality and structure of sperm, potentially causing birth defects.

While alcohol is a toxin, the body can handle a small amount of it. For most people, an occasional glass of wine at dinner or a cocktail at a social event does not appear to be harmful.

Coffee

More than 80 percent of Americans drink coffee. While some studies show benefits from drinking coffee, drinking more than a small amount of it is a bad idea. A 2013 study in the *Mayo Clinic Proceedings* found that in men under the age of fifty-five drinking four or more cups per day increases the risk of premature death by 56 percent.

YOUR MAINTENANCE LIST
FOR THE NUTRITION PATHWAY:
Foods to Avoid and the Reasons to Avoid Them

Energy Production

Avoid sugar. It binds with proteins to create advanced glycation end products (AGEs), damaging enzymes needed for energy production.

Fructose especially lowers energy levels.

Processed "supermarket" oils lower energy production.

Inflammation

Avoid sugar. It creates AGEs that cause inflammation.

Sugar increases insulin, which increases inflammation.

Avoid wheat. It quickly metabolizes to sugar and causes inflammation.

The gluten in wheat causes inflammation in the brain and throughout the body.

The lectins in wheat, even in small quantities, create inflammation.

Avoid supermarket oils. An excess of omega-6 oils leads to inflammation.

Avoid dairy. Immune reactions to milk protein cause inflammation.

Avoid glutamates. They are highly inflammatory.

Avoid GMO foods, such as soy and corn. They are inflammatory.

Acid/Alkaline Balance

Avoid sugar. It is acid-forming in the body.

Avoid Splenda. It raises the pH level in the intestines.

Avoid wheat. Immune reactions to gluten make the body more acidic.

Avoid dairy and meat products. They are acid-forming.

Avoid excess salt. It has an acidic effect.

Digestive Health

Avoid sugar. It interferes with the predigestive action of saliva and puts an extra burden on the pancreas, affecting the production of digestive enzymes.

Avoid dairy. Casein is difficult to digest and putrefies in the intestines, producing toxins.

Avoid GMO foods. The glyphosate they contain damages the digestive system.

Hormone Balance

Avoid sugar. It increases insulin and disrupts hormonal balance.

Fructose interferes with appetite-suppressing hormones, causing you to overeat.

Avoid supermarket oils. They interfere with hormonal balance.

Avoid wheat. The lectins disrupt hormones that regulate food consumption.

Avoid meat, milk, and dairy products. They are loaded with hormones that disrupt your hormonal balance.

Avoid excess animal protein. It disrupts hormonal balance by increasing estrogen levels in the body.

Avoid GMO foods. They contain hormone disrupting glyphosate (Roundup).

Platelet Stickiness

Avoid sugar. It causes platelet stickiness.

Avoid wheat. The lectins stimulate platelet stickiness.

Avoid excess salt. It promotes to platelet stickiness.

"Supermarket" oils promote platelet stickiness.

Fat Storage

Avoid high-fructose corn syrup. It interferes with appetite suppression.

Metabolized fructose results in fatty acids that get stored as fat.

Avoid sugar and grains. They increase insulin, which causes cells to store fat.

Avoid lectins. They block hormones that regulate food consumption and cause weight gain.

Avoid glutamates. They result in excess fat storage.

Cutting bad foods out of your life is one step; putting good foods in is another. Let's have a look at what we *should* be eating.

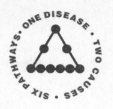

SIX

Choosing a Better Diet

*Y*ou are what you eat. Every cell in your body is made from what you eat and drink. Most of our health problems are the result of eating and drinking the wrong things. We are creating new cells that are defective because they were not built with the proper construction materials. Even if you constructed each new cell properly, you may not be supplying them with what they need to operate properly. This second of two Nutrition Pathway chapters will help you choose a better diet. *The key to good health is to eat a diet of primarily fresh, organically produced plant foods such as vegetables, fruits, nuts, seeds, legumes, sprouts, and a few whole grains, excluding wheat.*

Federal guidelines recommend nine servings of fruits and vegetables per day, yet only 10 percent of us do that. While no consensus exists on the perfect human diet, consider gorillas, who are close relatives with DNA similar to ours; they consume almost 100 percent of their calories from raw plants. Most of us consume less than 10 percent from raw plants, and many consume less than 5 percent.

The key to health is to make sure your cells are getting everything they need to be properly constructed and to do their jobs. Cells have a grocery list of essential nutrients that you must supply regularly. To keep yourself in good repair and biologically young, you have to deliver those groceries. Every day, you create hundreds of billions of new cells, and constructing them properly requires a bewildering array of complex chemicals. The construction materials to make these cells must come from your diet, but modern diets based on mineral depleted soils and filled with processed foods fail to supply these needs. The result is our epidemic of chronic disease and accelerated aging. By contrast, raw plant foods can supply a balance of proteins, carbohydrates, and oils, as well as the vitamins, minerals, phytochemicals, and fiber that we need. Eating unprocessed foods is essential. Fresh vegetables along with fruits, nuts, seeds, sprouts, and legumes must be the foundation of your diet.

Our genes are still those of our hunter-gatherer ancestors and require the same nutrition as they did back then. We are not getting that nutrition, and the result is our catastrophic epidemic of chronic disease and disability. Researchers estimate that the food our ancestors ate gave them about four times more nutrients than the food we eat today, and for certain nutrients that number is twenty or even fifty times higher. Yet because of the many changes in our environment and lifestyle, our need for nutrients is higher than ever—our intake of nutrients is down while our need is up. Most people are unaware of the unprecedented burden that our exposure to environmental toxins is placing on our bodies, dramatically increasing our need for nutrients. Meanwhile, most people choose foods for taste and convenience not nutrition. The concept of choosing foods for nutrition and health benefits is certainly not the norm in our society. Modern diets are overloaded with biologically inappropriate sugar, grains, dairy, salt, processed foods, GMO foods, and toxic food additives.

Hundreds of studies show that eating more fresh fruits and vegetables reduces the risk of all types of disease. For example, simply eating a diet of predominantly fruits and vegetables can cut your cancer risk by up to 75 percent. Fresh fruits and vegetables contain large amounts of phytochemicals, which are nature's way of protecting plants against disease and environmental stress. Phytochemicals give fruits and vegetables their brilliant colors, and they are primarily responsible for the disease-prevention capabilities of these healthy foods. By choosing a variety of fresh fruits and vegetables, you can provide your body with thousands of different phytochemicals that slow the aging process and offer enormous protection against all disease.

Eating more fruits and vegetables even decreases your appetite for processed foods. The best vegetables to keep the body biologically young and healthy are the cruciferous vegetables: cabbage, broccoli, kale, Brussels sprouts, turnips, cauliflower, radishes, bok choy, and watercress. Other good vegetables include carrots, onions, beets, and spinach. Good fruits include avocados, cherries, blackberries, blueberries, raspberries, pineapples, watermelon, kiwis, mangos, plums, and honeydew melons. Fruits are healthy, but consume them in moderation because of their high sugar content. Fruit juices should be avoided completely. The sugar is too bioavailable, rapidly increasing blood sugar and insulin. Orange juice with your breakfast is a bad choice!

The nutrients in vegetables can be made even more bioavailable by juicing or blenderizing. Using a juicer or powerful blender to mechanically break the tough cell walls of the plant releases more nutrition. In fact, you can get three times more nutrition from the same food than if you chewed it. Chewing makes only a fraction of the nutrition available. Making matters worse, most people don't chew well. A combination of juicing and blenderizing is best. Juicing is less filling because it removes the fiber, which allows you to consume more vegetables and get more nutrients. Blenderizing retains the fiber, and most of us don't get enough fiber. Many suitable juicers and blenders are on the market. Experiment with a variety of vegetables, and drink a glass of vegetable juice every day.

In addition to lots of fresh, raw vegetables, nongluten grains such as buckwheat, millet, brown rice, quinoa, and amaranth are okay in moderation, but grains are not a natural dietary choice for humans. Legumes and lentils are good sources of plant protein. Occasional small portions of high-quality animal protein, including organic eggs, can be added. Sprouts are an excellent food choice. However, store-bought sprouts are too often contaminated with bacteria and mold. Growing your own sprouts is best and simple to do. Sprouting is a fast, inexpensive way to produce high-quality food in your own kitchen.

Most of us are still eating the diet we grew up with, but if you want to be healthy, this behavior has to change. The best description for the Standard American Diet is "bizarre." No one in history has ever consumed such a diet. According to Department of Agriculture statistics, over the last century, average consumption of fresh apples declined by more than three-fourths, fresh cabbage by more than two-thirds, and fresh fruit by more than one-third. Historically unprecedented, the diet we are eating is incapable of supporting healthy life. Yet we feed this diet to our children! That's why, after accidents, cancer is now the leading cause of death for children, and diabetes, asthma, allergies, and cognitive/behavioral problems are epidemic.

Food Preparation

Ideally, at least 80 percent of your diet should be consumed raw. Cooking destroys nutrients and creates toxins. Eating the right foods is critical, but how you prepare those foods is also critical. Cooking food is a major change we have made in our diets, and it is an obstacle to meeting our bodies' nutritional needs. Cooking reduces the availability of many nutrients and phytochemicals. Cooking carrots, for example, can destroy 75 percent of vitamin C, 70 percent of B1, 50 percent of B2, and 60 percent of vitamin B3. Produce such as apples, beets, cabbage, and cauliflower lose most of their anticancer activity when they are cooked. The higher the heat and the longer the cooking time, the more nutrients are lost. If necessary, the best way to cook vegetables—for example, broccoli or spinach—is to lightly steam or quickly stir-fry them. Cooking food is a poor choice, yet we have elevated this mistake to an art form.

How you cook makes a difference. People in our society unfortunately love to eat fried and roasted foods. We love to caramelize (brown) our foods. We do this despite the research indicating that eating proteins, fats, and carbohydrates that have been cooked at high temperatures causes colon cancer. Cooking food at high temperatures, such as in grilling, frying, and barbecuing, destroys nutrients. High heat causes chemical reactions that make proteins less digestible, which results in more undigested proteins entering the colon. There, they are metabolized into a variety of toxic, cancer-causing waste products. This process helps to explain the association between colon cancer and diets rich in fried and roasted meats.

Cooking at high temperatures not only destroys nutrients, it also poisons the food by producing a variety of powerful toxins. The high heat of grilling causes reactions with the proteins in red meat, poultry, and fish, producing carcinogens such as heterocyclic amines, benzopyrenes, and polycyclic aromatic hydrocarbons. Meat that has been blackened is the worst of all. Never eat blackened meat or any blackened food. Even well-done meat is highly contaminated with carcinogens. Any time you cook meat at high temperatures, whether by barbecuing, frying, or broiling, carcinogens are created. When you cook meat, it is best to slow cook it at a low temperature, such as in a Crock-Pot. Especially avoid melted cheese, such as in pizza or a cheeseburger, as heated milk casein has been shown to be the most carcinogenic protein of all. Avoid all kinds of caramelized sugar, toasted bread, and roasted nuts. The bottom line: *All proteins cooked at high temperatures have been proven to cause cancer in laboratory animals, and numerous studies have shown that people who eat meat cooked at higher temperatures have more cancer.* Eating raw food is best.

Microwave ovens are found in almost every kitchen, yet *microwaving food is very dangerous.* It produces unique toxins and carcinogens that poison the body. In addition to creating toxins, microwaving causes massive destruction of nutrients. When cooked in a microwave, broccoli loses 97 percent of its antioxidants—only 11 percent is lost when steamed. Steaming is the least damaging way to cook.

Food Combining

What kind of foods you eat at the same meal is also important, particularly for older people or people already suffering from some chronic health problem. Many steps are involved in releasing the nutrients from the food you eat and then transporting these nutrients to the cells that need them. Proper digestion requires that a progressive series of processes go well in order to turn your food into vital nourishment. Otherwise, even the healthiest food can become toxic waste.

How you eat makes a difference. If you eat too fast or under stress, or if you eat the wrong combination of foods at a meal, the food may not be properly digested. *If the food isn't properly digested, you can't get the full nutritional value. Further, undigested food promotes the creation of dangerous toxins that poison the body.* The resulting deficiency and toxicity contribute to aging and disease.

Digestion begins in the mouth. Each stage in the process of digestion, from mouth to stomach to intestines, requires a specialized set of enzymes. Start the digestive process by chewing your food thoroughly, providing ample time to mix the enzymes with the food. Your pH is also important to this process. If your saliva pH is too acidic, these enzymes can become disabled.

Different food categories require different combinations of digestive juices for proper digestion. Proper *food combining* means eating those foods together that require the same chemical environment for their digestion. Proteins need a very acidic environment. Starchy foods, such as grains in any form (bread, pasta, rice, etc.) and potatoes, are digested in a more alkaline environment. If you eat both a starch and a protein at the same time, expect problems. Also, starches require less time in the stomach before moving on to the intestinal tract, where much of their digestion occurs. When starches enter the stomach along with proteins, which require a longer time there, they get held up. The starch begins to ferment, creating toxins and causing gas, bloating, abdominal discomfort, acid indigestion, poor nutrient absorption, and many other problems. Since most people in our society eat proteins and starches together (the meat-and-potatoes diet), indigestion and acid reflux have become normal. Americans spend more than $2 billion a year on antacids!

Fruits generally contain all of the enzymes necessary for their digestion, so they can and should pass through the system in much less time than either starch or protein. Some fruits, such as melons, are only in the stomach for fifteen to twenty minutes. Others are there slightly longer, but none as long as starch, let alone protein. When you eat a big meal and then have fruit for dessert, your stomach is already full and mixing in enzymes as it churns the meal. Along comes fruit, which is designed to pass right through, but now it cannot. It is stuck behind the meal. When fruit is forced to remain in the stomach with a starch, the mixture ferments and creates toxins that spread throughout the body. If the fruit remains in the stomach with a protein meal, digestion is again impaired, and the protein putrefies, similarly resulting in powerful toxins being released into your body.

Our digestive systems were not designed to eat what has become the "normal" diet of protein and starch meals. You can still enjoy these foods, but learning a new way to eat them will maximize the benefit you receive from them. If you eat three meals a day, have one fruit meal, one starch meal, and one protein meal (not necessarily animal protein). By digesting properly, you won't feel sleepy after meals because digesting the food will not take all the energy from your body. You'll feel energized because your body is not struggling with an impossible task and is able to actually use the nutrients, which your body has broken down and can now absorb. In addition, you will not be poisoned by fermentation by-products.

The common eating habits of our culture constantly create bad combinations for digestion. Most popular foods today are based upon poor food combinations—spaghetti and meatballs, chicken stir-fry over rice, pizza, hamburgers and French fries, any sandwich that contains meat, tacos, and even trail mixes that combine protein nuts, starchy grains, and dried fruit. You can make better choices by following these four guidelines:

- *Eat starches with vegetables*, but not with protein or fruit. Starches include grains, pasta, or bread, and starchy vegetables such as potatoes, sweet potato, corn, legumes, and beans.

- *Eat protein with nonstarchy vegetables*, and not with starches. Proteins include nuts, seeds, eggs, meat, or fish.
- *Eat fruit alone.* Sweet fruits should ideally be eaten after acid fruits, and acid fruits, such as citrus fruits, apples, mango, all berries, cherries, pears, apricots, and peaches may be eaten with raw nuts.
- *Melons should be eaten alone.*

Why Fiber Is Important

Fiber is the indigestible portion of plant foods that nevertheless plays a vital role in human digestion. Soluble fiber produces food for the cells lining the gut and supports friendly bacteria in the colon. Insoluble fiber aids in elimination, shortening the time it takes for the undigested food particles and toxins to pass through the intestinal tract. Fiber helps to normalize the body's insulin levels. In addition, fresh foods that are high in fiber are also high in nutrition, including the carotenes, flavonoids, and antioxidants that are known to help prevent and reverse disease. Good fiber sources include kidney beans, garbanzo beans, navy beans, whole grains, legumes, and raw vegetables. Although fiber is very important, it is lacking in our diets. Many nutritional experts recommend 35 to 45 grams (g) of fiber per day. The average American gets about 15 g.

The Choice Is Simple

Human nutrition is extremely complex, but the choice that we need to make is simple. Either we continue to think of foods as entertainment and eat foods that make us sick, or we think of food as building materials for our cells and eat foods that make us healthy. Cells are chemical factories. More than 100,000 chemical reactions take place in each cell every second, producing thousands and thousands of chemicals that you need to stay alive and function. The raw materials for these chemical reactions come from the food you eat.

A chronic shortage of even one essential nutrient affects the entire system and causes disease. You need to be mindful of everything you put in your mouth. Every mouthful should supply the most nutrition for the least number of calories, and we have to train ourselves to think about food this way. To get the nutrition you need, you have to eat real food with the highest nutrient density. Real food is what nature provides—naturally ripened, freshly harvested, unprocessed, and loaded with nutrition. Unfortunately, real food is now in short supply—some people eat almost no real food at all. What they eat may be called "food" and may look like food, but it is not fit to eat and it is making them sick. Modern processed foods are deficient in nutrients and high in toxins. They cause disease. Even most of the so-called fresh foods are weeks to months old by the time you get them and have lost most of their nutritional value. For these reasons, the Standard American Diet does not support healthy life.

As much as possible, follow these rules:

- Eat a diet of primarily fresh plant foods.
- Avoid processed foods.
- Eat 80 percent of your diet raw.
- Eat primarily organic foods.
- Juice or blenderize fresh vegetables every day.
- Be wary of restaurant foods, unless organic and raw.
- Avoid processed, supermarket fats and oils.
- Get on a high-quality supplement program.
- Consume a balance of healthy omega-6 and omega-3 oils.
- Include high-quality flaxseed, coconut, and olive oils in your diet.
- Avoid sugar and wheat, and minimize grains.
- Avoid dairy products.

- Limit alcohol and coffee.
- Avoid foods high in mold, such as peanuts, corn, and dried fruits.
- Avoid barbecued and microwaved foods.
- Minimize animal protein, and it must be organic and not grain fed.

Supplements

Supplements have become a necessity. According to the National Academy of Sciences, *even if you eat a good diet, it is no longer possible to get all the nutrition you need for good health.* While human genes have survived almost unchanged since prehistoric times, the prehistoric diet has not. Our soils are depleted of nutrients. The original varieties of many fruits and vegetables have become extinct. Our farmed animals are just as sick and nutrient deficient as the rest of the food chain. The reality is this: The food we eat today is far less nutritious than the food we were eating just fifty years ago. Unless you live in extraordinary circumstances, you simply cannot get all the nutrition you need from food alone—even if you eat a good diet with lots of fresh fruits and vegetables. You have to compensate for these deficiencies by supplementing.

You Can No Longer Get All the Nutrition You Need from Food Alone

A key aspect of healthy eating is choosing foods that have not been adulterated. Eating foods that are as close as possible to their natural state is the only way to get the maximum amount of the nutrients that are found in fresh, raw foods. However, today's food supply is enormously compromised. The combination of modern chemical farming, harvesting before ripening, processing, pasteurizing, irradiating, storing, and shipping has reduced the nutritional quality of our food to the point where it can no longer support healthy life. To begin, farming with artificial fertilizers does not replace minerals in the soil. Pesticides and herbicides destroy beneficial bacteria and earthworms that transform inorganic minerals in the soil into organically available minerals that plants can take up into their roots. Monoculture farming—planting the same crops year after year, without resting the field or rotating the crops—further depletes the soil. Our soils are now stripped of essential minerals, and almost all of us are mineral deficient.

Another reason modern produce is nutrient poor is the practice of harvesting crops before they are ripe. This helps get the food to you before it rots but reduces its nutritional content by up to 80 percent because much of the nutrition develops in the last day or two of ripening. Then there is the problem of distribution. Food is best harvested when ripe and consumed shortly thereafter. With each passing hour after harvest, nutrition is lost. Significantly the average age of produce in the supermarket is two weeks, and some items are more than a year old. "Fresh" apples average about ten months old and are often more than a year old. They may still look like apples, but they have little nutritional value. Studies on "fresh" oranges have found that many contain no vitamin C whatsoever. These so-called fresh oranges are harvested green, stored in warehouses, artificially colored, and sold as fresh.

Food is hardy, but nutrients are not. Nutrients are easily lost or destroyed. For example, spinach loses 60 percent of its folic acid in three days. Vegetables such as asparagus, broccoli, and green beans lose 50 percent of their vitamin C before they reach the produce section. Cooking these vegetables results in even more losses, including another 25 percent of the vitamin C, 70 percent of vitamin B1, and 50 percent of B2.

The nutritional content of every vegetable grown in the United States has undergone huge declines. A 2001 study in the *Nutrition Practitioner* looked at mineral levels in food over a fifty-year period. The study found that to get the same amount of calcium you received from one carrot half a century ago, you now have to eat two carrots. It takes four carrots to get the same magnesium, and up to twenty carrots to get the same amount of zinc. In 1940, one cup of spinach supplied 80 mg of iron. Today it would take sixty-seven cups to get the same amount. Iron deficiency increases the stickiness of blood platelets, causing strokes in children and adults. No one is eating all these extra vegetables! This is why most adult women don't get even the RDA for calcium, magnesium, zinc, the B vitamins, and vitamin E. Half of all Americans over age sixty are deficient in vitamins A, C, and E.

Severe deficiencies of vitamins and minerals are uncommon in developed nations, but modest deficiencies are the norm. Perhaps a modest deficiency doesn't sound so bad, but remember that to do its job of repairing your cells and keeping you biologically young and healthy, the body must have *everything* it needs. A chronic shortage of even one essential nutrient throws the entire body out of balance. Consider when a tiny gear is missing from an expensive watch. No matter how expensive the watch, it will not keep good time. A 2011 study published in the *FASEB Journal* found that even moderate deficiencies of selenium and vitamin K impair normal cell functions that over time cause so-called age-related diseases. Once you get sick, your doctor will blame your age, but really your diet is at fault.

Unfortunately, you can no longer get sufficient amounts of certain vitamins and minerals from your diet. Although whole food should still be your main source of nutrition, supplementation is required to make sure your cells are getting everything they need. Vitamin and mineral supplements are essential and remarkably safe. But I'll be the first to admit that it is difficult to find brands that do what they are supposed to do and deliver high-quality, bioavailable nutrients. Nevertheless, it is possible to make them, and that is why I designed my own high-quality Beyond Health brand supplements. While the need for specific nutrients varies greatly according to a person's condition and unique biochemistry, I cover in this chapter a few of the most common deficiencies and supplements.

Let's have a look at what some nutritional supplements can do for you.

Multivitamins Make for Younger Cells

Taking a multivitamin is a good way to ensure that your body is getting a steady supply of essential nutrients. A 2009 study in the *American Journal of Clinical Nutrition* compared the biological age (telomere length) of the cells of people who took multivitamins and those who did not. Those taking a multivitamin every day were biologically younger and aging slower.

CoQ10

CoQ10 is a critical cofactor in mitochondrial energy production. A coenzyme Q10 deficiency can lead to sluggish thinking and memory decline. People with high levels of CoQ10 have been proven in studies to have better motor abilities, higher mental acuity, and increased energy production. It also reduces the symptoms and progression of neurodegenerative diseases such as Alzheimer's. Supplementation is important because our ability to produce CoQ10 declines as we age.

Zinc

Are you one of the 70 percent of Americans who, according to the USDA, aren't getting the Recommended Daily Intake (RDI) of zinc? Or could you be getting the RDI, but still not enough for optimal health?

Zinc is a key element in regulating cellular aging, but if you're not getting enough, accelerated aging is only one of a host of problems you're likely to face. Apart from its well-known role in immunity, zinc is required for the activity of more than 300 different enzymes and is involved in most major metabolic pathways. Here are just some of the reasons you may want to make sure you're getting enough zinc from food and supplements:

- Zinc supports immunity and is crucial for thymus gland and T-cell function. Taking zinc within twenty-four hours of getting a cold can shorten the length of time you'll have the cold and reduce the severity of symptoms.

- Older people with normal levels of zinc are half as likely to get pneumonia as those who are deficient. As we age, we need more zinc to maintain immunity, but our ability to absorb it decreases. As a result, zinc levels are often low among the elderly.

- Zinc protects against cancer. A 2011 study in *Cancer Biology and Therapy* found zinc to suppress pancreatic cancer tumors. Other studies have found that zinc slows the development of prostate cancer.

- Zinc helps to prevent osteoporosis. It is necessary for normal bone synthesis, and studies show that older people with osteoporosis test low on zinc.

- Zinc is essential for healthy skin. It is used in treating acne, eczema, and other skin diseases.

- Zinc supports eye health. It is the most abundant mineral in the eyes. Studies show that zinc protects against macular degeneration and resulting vision loss.

- Zinc supports fertility. Men and women both need adequate zinc levels for reproduction, and zinc is often used to treat infertility.

- Zinc supports the senses. Two symptoms of zinc deficiency are diminished taste acuity and diminished sense of smell.

- Zinc is highest in the protein-rich foods, particularly shellfish (especially oysters), but also in meat, poultry, and liver. Additional good sources of zinc are pumpkin and sunflower seeds, pecans, oats, and eggs. To maintain top immunity, supplementing with 30 mg of zinc per day is recommended.

Magnesium: One of the Hardest-Working Minerals in the Body

About 70 percent of Americans do not consume the recommended daily intake of magnesium, and more than 80 percent of our elderly do not. Magnesium is the fourth most abundant mineral in the body, and it is involved in more than 300 types of biochemical reactions in the body. It helps maintain normal muscle and nerve function, keeps heart rhythm steady, supports a healthy immune system, and keeps bones strong. Magnesium also helps to regulate blood sugar levels, promote normal blood pressure, and support energy production and protein synthesis. Any shortage of magnesium will result in multiple dysfunctions.

Magnesium deficiency is associated with most diseases attributed to old age, including arthritis, Alzheimer's, cancer, diabetes, stroke, heart disease, hypertension, osteoporosis, insomnia, and thyroid disorders. Telomerase is an enzyme that repairs telomeres, but telomerase synthesis is dependent on the amount of magnesium available. Thus, a shortage of magnesium results in telomere shortening and aging.

Magnesium is absolutely essential to oxygen respiration. It is involved in every single step in the production of energy in normal cells, yet most of us are deficient in this mineral. Magnesium deficiency causes cells to switch energy production to fermentation, which produces much less energy, more acid, and many dangerous free radicals. Older adults are at a particular risk for magnesium deficiency. In aged individuals, magnesium absorption decreases and renal excretion of magnesium increases.

Older adults are also more likely to be taking drugs that interact with magnesium. Virtually everyone should be taking a high-quality magnesium supplement.

The digestive tract does not absorb magnesium easily; only about 50 percent of magnesium in foods is absorbed. If you have digestive problems, such as a leaky gut and food allergies, you absorb even less. Even people with a healthy gut who eat a high-magnesium diet with magnesium-rich vegetables, whole grains, nuts, and seeds may not be able to rely upon food alone to provide sufficient magnesium because our soils are so depleted. Mercury fillings and other forms of exposure to mercury prevent the body from absorbing and using magnesium. Fluoride also binds with magnesium and prevents absorption.

Drinking caffeine, carbonated soft drinks, and alcohol wastes magnesium. Eating a lot of dairy products and other foods high in calcium can also affect magnesium levels. So does eating sugar. A number of drugs interfere with magnesium absorption and utilization, including the birth control pill, antibiotics, antihistamines, and aspirin. Finally yet importantly, stress uses a lot of magnesium. If you are under stress, you need more magnesium.

Selenium

We obtain antioxidants from food and supplements, but the body also makes powerful antioxidants. By far, the most important of these is glutathione. Glutathione cannot be made without the enzyme glutathione peroxidase, which in turn cannot be made without selenium. When selenium is in short supply, the lack of this critical enzyme results in cancer, heart disease, arthritis, aging, and loss of immunity and brain functioning.

Selenium helps protect the brain from aging. Our environment has a lot of mercury in it, and a toxic form of mercury—methylmercury—accumulates in the brain and damages the nervous system. Selenium helps to neutralize methylmercury. Selenium blood levels drop with age; supplementation is usually needed.

B Vitamins Increase Energy

The benefits of B vitamins are truly amazing. B vitamins work together as a team and are essential to a multitude of functions in the body, including energy production. You need to get the whole team. Yet B vitamin deficiencies are among the most common deficiencies, and an estimated 40 percent of the U.S. population is B12 deficient. One problem is that only the highest-quality supplements contain the most biologically active forms of B vitamins, such as the pyridoxal 5-phosphate form of vitamin B6. As you age, the need for B vitamins increases. Muscles start to deteriorate after age thirty, but a combination of regular exercise and B vitamins can actually reverse this process. Vitamin B6 is important for healthy brain function and mental clarity. Vitamin B3 is critical for maintaining the body's energy levels. Vitamin B12 slows down telomere degradation. A B12 deficiency can cause symptoms of aging, including cognitive problems and poor memory, muscle weakness, fatigue, shakiness, unsteady gait, low blood pressure, mood disorders, and depression. Unfortunately, most B12 supplements are in the form of cyanocobalamin, a cheap and biologically inappropriate form of B12.

Vitamin C: The King of Vitamins

Vitamin C is one of the most powerful vitamins you can take. Most people don't get enough of this youth-enhancing, antiaging vitamin, which stabilizes blood pressure, boosts the immune system, fights colds and flu, and is an outstanding cancer fighter. It is a powerful antioxidant that neutralizes free radicals produced in the body. Vitamin C retards telomere shortening, slowing the aging process. It is also necessary for synthesizing collagen, the most important protein for maintaining elasticity and strength of the skin, arteries, and other body tissues. Vitamin C is your best defense against aging and wrinkles. Most adults should supplement with 6,000 mg per day in divided doses, and more if suffering from a chronic disease.

Vitamin D: Both a Hormone and a Nutrient

Vitamin D affects so many body functions, getting adequate amounts is critical. Yet between 40 to 75 percent of the teen and adult population is deficient, more in the winter and less in the summer. Vitamin D is essential to calcium metabolism, supports bone health, helps to control blood sugar, supports immunity, and protects against cancer. Vitamin D significantly increases the production of telomerase, the enzyme that repairs telomeres, which helps keep your telomeres long, slows aging, and keeps you biologically young.

Vitamin D plays an important role in muscle function, and low levels reduce muscle strength and physical performance. According to data from the National Institute on Aging, older adults who have trouble walking several blocks or climbing a flight of stairs may be deficient in vitamin D. Low vitamin D levels have also been linked to diabetes, hypertension, cardiovascular disease, and lung disease—conditions that frequently cause decline in physical function.

It's difficult to get enough vitamin D through diet alone. The best source is exposure to sunlight, and if you do not spend enough time outdoors, you need to supplement. Many researchers recommend 5,000 to 10,000 IU per day. Measuring vitamin D is easy with a blood test, and you should keep your vitamin D level at the upper end of the normal range—above 50 ng/ml (nanograms per milliliter).

Vitamin E: A Powerful Antioxidant

About 30 percent of the U.S. population is vitamin E deficient. Vitamin E protects against oxidative damage to tissues. A powerful antioxidant, vitamin E helps prevent cellular aging by neutralizing free radicals that can lead to genetic mutations and tissue damage. Vitamin E retards telomere shortening, slowing the aging process, and supports immunity. Supplement with 400 to 800 IU per day.

Acetyl L-Carnitine and Lipoic Acid

Damage to mitochondria (the energy-producing powerhouses of the cell) is a major contributor to aging and associated degenerative diseases. Lipoic acid is a powerful antioxidant compound that protects the mitochondria from damage and supports energy production while offering protection from age-related memory decline and strokes. Acetyl L-carnitine supports energy production by transporting fatty acid fuel into the mitochondria and supporting normal oxygen respiration in the cell. In higher doses, these two supplements work together synergistically and appear to reverse much of the decay process due to aging and to improve brain and other functions by rejuvenating the mitochondria.

Curcumin

Curcumin is a component of the spice turmeric. It works well for many inflammation-driven conditions, and it reduces edema. It lowers cholesterol and triglyceride levels, helps to prevent heart disease by inhibiting inflammation and oxidative damage, and prevents blood clots by inhibiting platelet aggregation. Curcumin can stop the buildup of the destructive beta-amyloid protein in the brain. Alzheimer's rates in India are among the lowest in the world, and research shows that curcumin is responsible.

Supplementation Is Essential

Until we start eating for nutrition and taking high-quality supplements, our epidemic of premature aging and chronic disease will continue. If you have a diagnosable disease, you are certainly suffering from multiple nutritional deficiencies. To overcome these deficiencies, changing your diet and taking high-quality supplements is essential.

Nobel Prize–winner Dr. Linus Pauling once said, "You can trace every sickness, every disease, and every ailment to a mineral deficiency." Yet the mineral content of our farm soils has decreased dramatically, especially over the last fifty years. Combine that with the mineral losses from food processing, and the result is that almost every American is mineral-deficient. No wonder more than three out of four Americans have a diagnosable chronic disease. You may have no symptoms, but if you consume foods that have little nutritional value or are toxic, you are almost certainly in the early stages of disease. The only way to end our chronic disease epidemic is to eat fresh, whole foods and supplement with high-quality supplements.

Health is a choice. The challenge is to choose it. Remember: *Nothing tastes as good as good health feels.*

Getting Back to Basics

To keep yourself at the highest level of health, you must consume a diet that Mother Nature intended you to eat. The consumption of processed foods must be kept to a minimum. As a simple guideline, be suspicious of any food product with an ingredients label. Thousands of studies show that eating a raw plant-based diet is dramatically protective against all diseases. Such a diet includes fresh vegetables and fruits, nuts, seeds, and sprouted foods. Foods such as beans, lentils, vegetables, apples, avocados, raw spinach, steamed broccoli, and whole grains contain soluble fiber that provides many health benefits. Cooking more than a small percentage of your food increases the risk of disease because cooking makes food less nutritious and deprives your cells of what they need to operate normally and keep you healthy.

YOUR MAINTENANCE LIST FOR THE NUTRITION PATHWAY: Food Combining, Supplements, and Digestive Health

Energy Production

Follow food combining rules to enable nutrients to be used for energy.

Take nutritional supplements that support energy production.

CoQ10 is a critical cofactor in mitochondrial energy production.

Magnesium is essential to every step in the production of energy.

B vitamins are critical for maintaining the body's energy levels.

Acetyl L-carnitine transports fatty acids to the mitochondria for fuel.

Lipoic acid is an antioxidant that protects mitochondria from damage.

Inflammation

Get plenty of antioxidants to reduce inflammation and preserve telomere length.

Supplement with curcumin, it inhibits inflammation and oxidative damage.

Supplement with selenium to assure adequate supplies of the antioxidant glutathione.

Acid/Alkaline Balance

Follow food combining rules to avoid acidity in the body.

Supplement with magnesium to support oxygen respiration in cells, preventing acid-forming fermentation.

Digestive Health

Chew thoroughly to give enzymes in saliva time to begin breaking down foods.

Do not impair digestion by eating too fast or when under stress.

Do not cook proteins at high heat because it makes them less digestible.

Avoid eating starch with protein because the starches ferment and the proteins putrefy.

Eat fruits by themselves, since they have their own enzymes and digest quickly.

Eat fiber because it supports friendly bacteria in the colon and helps with elimination.

Hormonal Balance

Take zinc to help control acne-related hormones.

Platelet Stickiness

Take curcumin to inhibit platelet aggregation and prevent blood clots.

Iron deficiency causes platelet stickiness—make sure your iron is in the normal range.

Fat Storage

Eat fresh, raw, whole plant foods and take high-quality supplements to eliminate excessive fat storage.

Eat fiber because it normalizes insulin levels, thus avoiding fat storage.

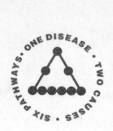

ONE DISEASE · TWO CAUSES · SIX PATHWAYS

SEVEN

Toxins Cause Disease

*As the first generation of man exposed to an
unprecedented plethora of daily chemicals, we have
learned that stored chemicals can mimic any disease.
"Incurable" chronic diseases that were thought
to have no known cause often disappear
when toxic chemicals are gone.*

—Sherry Rogers, M.D., author of *Tired or Toxic?*

*Our health is threatened not only by
individual chemicals—deadly or toxic—
but even more by the overall chemical load that
the human organism now has to sustain.*

—Joseph D. Beasley, M.D., Ph.D., *The Kellogg Report*

*The greatest part of all chronic disease is
created by . . . drug poisoning.*

—Henry Lindlahr, M.D.

*T*oxicity is one of the two causes of all disease. Today we are living in a chemically based society, and *almost all of us are in toxic overload.* These toxins are a major cause of our chronic disease epidemic. That's the bad news. The good news is that you can learn how to reduce your load to manageable levels. This Toxin Pathway chapter tells you how to avoid toxins and how to reduce your toxic load.

Never before in history has the human organism been exposed to so many toxins. Our bodies are not designed to protect themselves from such an overwhelming onslaught of man-made chemicals, and these chemicals are bioaccumulating inside us. Our toxic overload, along with our poor diets, is directly responsible for our epidemic of chronic disease as well as the many mystery syndromes that are products of the late twentieth century, such as chronic fatigue, fibromyalgia, and chemical sensitivity. Toxins affect all of your maintenance systems. They depress energy production, cause inflammation, damage digestion, disrupt hormonal balance, promote platelet stickiness, and cause overweight.

Americans are bioaccumulating hundreds of man-made chemicals in their bodies, yet few are aware this is happening and of the effects these chemicals are having on our health. Making matters worse, our physicians are oblivious to this reality; they rarely test for toxins. In fact, physicians are major contributors to our toxic overloads through their use of toxic vaccines and prescription drugs. A number of researchers believe that aging is a slow poisoning resulting from a lifetime accumulation of toxins in the body. With tens of thousands of man-made chemicals in our environment, we have all become toxic dump sites.

Toxic Planet, Toxic People

In her book *Toxic Overload*, Paula Baillie-Hamilton, M.D., had this to say: "We are now one of the most polluted species on the face of this planet. . . . Indeed, we are all so contaminated that if we were cannibals our meat would be banned from human consumption." The air we breathe, the foods we eat, the water we drink, and even everyday products such as clothing, toothpaste, and the lotions we put on our skin—all expose us to toxic chemicals that interfere with normal cell function. We live in a toxic world, and each year our world is becoming even more toxic. As a result, most of us are accumulating toxins faster than we can get rid of them.

We get sicker as we get older because we become progressively more toxic. For the last century, mankind has been unwittingly involved in a vast and complex experiment in chemical living. We live in a sea of toxins, and we now know that this is having a catastrophic effect on our health, interfering with vital biologic processes and causing our cells and systems to malfunction. Yet this experiment not only continues; it is expanding. The toxins accumulating in our bodies are causing massive cellular malfunction, even in the unborn. A study presented at the American Heart Association's Scientific Sessions 2013 concluded that heart defects in newborns are closely associated with their mother's exposure to environmental toxins during pregnancy. The same holds for many of the other health problems we are seeing in our children. Significant evidence now shows that exposure to environmental toxins before conception and during pregnancy cause miscarriages, stillbirth, premature birth, birth defects, childhood cancers, and cognitive impairment.

Annoying symptoms like headaches, insomnia, gastrointestinal disturbances, joint and muscle pain, allergies, increased pulse rate, and high blood pressure—plus serious debilitating conditions like heart disease, cancer, immune disorders, endocrine disorders, and many more—can be caused by environmental toxins. These toxins also disrupt neurotransmitters in the brain and the nervous system, giving rise to anxiety, depression, fatigue, hyperactivity, and even violent behavior. They also drive disorders like Alzheimer's, Parkinson's, and autism.

Resistance to disease plummets as toxins build up in our bodies. By retirement age, our accumulated toxic loads are more than sufficient to cause cancer. To make matters worse, the detoxification capacity of our kidneys and liver diminishes with age, further challenging our older population, who already have the highest concentrations of toxic chemicals. Contributing even more to this toxic overload, most of our older people are on prescription drugs. Drugs add substantially to their toxic burden, causing fatigue, poor memory, disorientation, and even death.

The threat to our health comes not only from individual chemicals but from the total chemical load we are sustaining and the interactions of the hundreds of chemicals stored in our tissues. Certain chemicals in combination become thousands of times more toxic than any one acting alone. For example, both arsenic and estrogen at high doses are known to cause cancer. However, these two acting together will cause cancer, even at low doses thought to be safe. Certain food additives, which alone do not harm test animals, will kill them when fed to them in combination. A big problem is that chemicals are tested for safety one at a time, yet we are exposed to them in combination. Babies are being born loaded with toxins acquired from their mothers, causing an epidemic of birth defects, hyperactivity disorders, learning disabilities, and childhood cancer. It's scary that almost nothing is known about the toxicity of the millions of possible combinations of these various chemicals and their carcinogenicity under various circumstances.

Given the magnitude of the problem, it may surprise you to learn that, according to the National Academy of Sciences, less than 10 percent of the nearly 80,000 chemicals used in commerce today have been tested for their capacity to cause cancer or do other damage to your health. Comparisons of cancer tissues with healthy tissues show that cancer tissues have a much higher concentration of toxic chemicals. We are told that our daily exposure to each is very small and not dangerous. However, daily exposure to even small amounts of thousands of toxic chemicals adds up over time, accumulating in your tissues to dangerous levels.

In 2009 the Centers for Disease Control and Prevention (CDC) published its *Fourth National Report on Human Exposure to Environmental Chemicals*, which tested for 212 chemicals. All 212 were found to be in the blood and urine of most Americans. Six highly toxic chemicals were found in virtually every person, including mercury and bisphenol-A, both of which are highly damaging, even in extremely small amounts.

What You Need to Do

A toxin is any substance that interferes with normal cellular function. Toxins can affect us in numerous ways. Some toxins, such as heavy metals like lead and mercury, shut down enzymes, making them unable to produce all the critical molecules we need, including antibodies, digestive enzymes, high-energy compounds, and hormones. Some toxins mimic hormones and give false signals to cells and genes, increasing the risk of hormone-dependent cancers. Others inhibit cell-to-cell communications, interfering with the body's ability to self-regulate. Some toxins directly damage DNA, causing mutations, while others react with DNA and change how genes express; both actions reprogram the cell's control system. Programming errors can lead to uncontrolled cell multiplication. Some toxins interfere with oxygen transport, while others damage immunity. The resulting malfunctions throw our chemistry out of balance, and *our bodies cease to effectively communicate, self-regulate, and self-repair.* This is disease!

The body is able to cope with toxins to a certain point; then you get sick. Our toxic overload combined with our nutrient deficiencies creates a devastating synergy. Constant exposure to tens of thousands of chemicals, from before birth onward, leads to the creation of excessive free radicals that cause disease of every description. Fortunately, you can take three actions to reduce the impact of toxins on your health:

- Reduce your exposure to toxins.
- Support your detoxification systems with nutrients.
- Reduce your burden of stored toxins.

Reduce Your Exposure:
Stop Putting Toxins In

We now live in a sea of chemicals to which we are exposed every moment of every day. They are in the air we breathe, the water we drink, and the food we eat. They are in our toothpaste, shampoo, cosmetics, cars, clothes, newspapers, magazines, furniture, and the prescription and over-the-counter drugs we take. These chemicals affect every cell in the body. We don't realize how many toxins bombard us every day because we can't see them. Even very small amounts of toxins can be devastating to your health. Yet more than 3,000 chemicals are added to our food. More than 700 chemicals can be found in city drinking water, including many prescription drugs. Americans are being exposed to tap water containing antibiotics, sleeping pills, sex hormones, and antidepressants. All these add up over time. According to EPA statistics, over a billion pounds of pesticides are used in the United States every year, and a percentage of that ends up in our bodies. The oceans are now so contaminated that it is unsafe to eat more than a very small quantity of fish.

Fortunately, we have personal control over most of our toxic exposures, and if we exercise that control, we can reduce our toxic overload to manageable levels. The body has the capacity to detoxify, but we are overloading it. Learning the sources of toxins and avoiding them are the first steps toward reducing your toxic overload.

In most cases, safe products can easily replace dangerous products. For example, eat organically produced foods. Choose to use safe household cleaning products, personal care products, pillows, mattresses, carpets, building materials, and paints. Use air filters and water filters in your home. Avoid prescription drugs. By making simple lifestyle choices, you can reduce your toxic load by an estimated 80 percent.

What's in Your Food?

To reduce your toxic load, start with the foods you eat. Almost any food you purchase in a supermarket is contaminated with multiple toxic chemicals.

As much as possible, avoid processed foods and eat fresh, organically produced foods. To the extent possible, purchase fresh foods at farmers' markets and food coops. Unfortunately, most people do not have a reliable supply of high-quality organic foods. As a practical matter, this means selecting from among the least toxic options in order to minimize the amount of toxins you consume. For example, bisphenol-A (BPA) is found in plastic water bottles. Eliminate your consumption of water packaged in plastic bottles—choose water packaged in glass bottles. Bisphenol-A is also found in almost all canned foods and beverages, and consumption of sodas has been linked to higher BPA levels in teenagers;

avoid canned foods and beverages. Minimize fish consumption. Mercury, present in fish as well as other sources such as dental fillings, causes cognitive dysfunction along with many other disease problems. Mercury damages the brain, and people with high mercury test lower for complex information processing. A 2012 study in *Integrative Medicine* found that people who eat the most fish have the most mercury in their systems.

Some of the most common food additives to avoid are benzoates, nitrites, nitrates, and glutamates. Doing this is simple—avoid processed foods. Meat, dairy products, and fish are contaminated with insecticides, fungicides, weed killers, hormones, antibiotics, prescription drugs, industrial chemicals, PCBs, dioxins, flame retardants, and heavy metals. About 90 percent of human exposure to many of these toxic contaminants comes from eating processed foods. Reduce your toxic exposure by eating only small quantities of organic meat, very limited quantities of fish, and eliminating milk and milk products from your diet.

The United States is the world's largest user of pesticides, using over one billion pounds per year. Pesticides bioaccumulate in cells and tissues, disrupt normal cell function, and cause every kind of disease. These toxic chemicals are found in fruits, vegetables, meat, dairy, and even tap water. People with high exposure to pesticides have high rates of cancer and neurological diseases. *Your exposure to pesticides can be cut by about 80 percent simply by switching to organic foods.* When you can achieve an 80 percent reduction so easily, what may have appeared as an impossible task suddenly becomes quite doable.

More than 70 percent of fruits and vegetables contain pesticide residues, which begin to accumulate in us at an early age, eventually reaching concentrations that cause major cellular malfunction and disease. The combined effects of multiple pesticides acting together can greatly magnify the effects of any of them acting alone. The U.S. Department of Agriculture admits that most of our pesticide load comes from meat and dairy products. The reason is that standards for animal feed are much less stringent than for humans. Their feed can be loaded with pesticides, and these chemicals become concentrated in their meat, ending up in our bodies. Do not use pesticides in your home or garden. Many safe alternatives are available. If you must use a pesticide around your home, garden, or office, use a safe, natural insecticide product like Orange Guard.

When forced to purchase nonorganic produce, know which is the safest. For a variety of reasons, certain produce is less heavily sprayed with pesticides than others. Following is a list of produce that is generally the least contaminated:

- Asparagus
- Avocados
- Cabbage
- Cantaloupe
- Cauliflower
- Eggplant
- Grapefruit
- Kiwi
- Mangoes
- Onions
- Papayas (Hawaiian papayas are GMO and should be avoided)
- Pineapples
- Sweet corn (American corn is a GMO and should be avoided)
- Sweet peas, frozen
- Sweet potatoes

On the other hand, here is a list of produce that you *should* buy organic because these foods are the most contaminated:

- Apples
- Blueberries (domestic)
- Celery
- Cherry tomatoes
- Cucumbers
- Grapes
- Hot peppers
- Lettuce
- Nectarines (imported)
- Peaches
- Potatoes
- Snap peas (imported)
- Spinach
- Strawberries
- Sweet bell peppers

Many people ask if eating organic foods really makes a difference. A 2003 study in *Environmental Health Perspectives* provides the answer. One group of children was fed a diet that was 75 percent organic foods, while another group was fed 75 percent conventional foods. The children's urine was then measured for pesticides. The children eating conventional foods measured four times the official safety limit. Yet after only a few days, the children in the organic group measured only one-sixth as much as the conventional group and within the safety limit. *Eating organic does make a difference—a big difference.*

Eliminating all processed foods is best. Not only are they deficient in nutrition, they are loaded with toxins. Flame retardants are found in dairy products, meat products, and farmed salmon. Milk is a toxic soup filled with pesticides, antibiotics, dioxins, hormones, sulfa drugs, tranquilizers, and other contaminants. Bread is often contaminated with potassium bromate, used as a dough conditioner. Bromate competes with iodine in the thyroid, causing thyroid malfunction. Commercial peanut butter is loaded with toxic chemical residues. According to the 1982–1986 FDA Total Diet Study, peanut butter had a whopping 183 residues. Frozen French fries contained seventy different pesticide residues. Frozen pizzas had sixty-seven industrial chemical and pesticide residues. Frozen chocolate cake contained sixty-one toxic residues, and milk chocolate had ninety-three. Caramel coloring is used in cola drinks and numerous other products, but it is not safe. During the production of caramel coloring, a carcinogenic byproduct, 4-methylimidazole, is created and remains in the product. All these toxins accumulate in your body, exaggerate each others' impact, and systematically destroy your health.

Of special concern are processed meats—such as sliced deli meats, bacon, ham, hot dogs, jerky, pastrami, pepperoni, salami, corned beef, and some sausages. These substantially increase the risk of bladder, colorectal, and pancreatic cancer. Eating just one serving of processed meat per day, such as a hot dog, sausage, or a few pieces of bacon, can increase your risk of premature death by over 20 percent. Techniques such as salting, smoking, and added chemicals are used to preserve the meat, prolong shelf life, inhibit bacterial growth, and enhance flavors. Smoking creates carcinogenic polycyclic aromatic hydrocarbons, which contaminate the meat. Nitrite preservatives are added to these meats to prevent bacterial growth and to help maintain color. Unfortunately, in the human body, these nitrite preservatives can be converted into compounds called *nitrosamines*, which are known carcinogens. *No amount of processed meat is safe, and no one should eat processed meats.*

Packaging materials (such as plastic wrap, plastic bottles, milk containers, juice boxes, Styrofoam, and epoxy can linings) can leach toxins into our foods before we eat them. Portions of the polymers, plasticizers, stabilizers, fillers, and colorants in plastic wrap can dissolve into the food. Even the wax paper used to package breakfast cereals has been found to leach toxic chemicals into the cereal. Ironically, people who are careful to buy organic foods may overlook the fact that they sometimes come in toxic packaging. Why purchase organic meat in a Styrofoam tray topped with plastic shrink-wrap, or organic canned goods in an epoxy-lined can?

What's in Your Water?

In December 2009 the *New York Times* published an analysis finding that during the previous five years, more than 20 percent of the water treatment systems in the United States had violated the safety standards in the Safe Drinking Water Act. The *Times* found that about 50 million Americans had been drinking water with unsafe levels of toxic chemicals, including arsenic, tetrachloroethylene, uranium, prescription drugs, and dangerous bacteria found in sewage. Meanwhile, several studies in the *American Journal of Epidemiology* indicate that negative health effects from these chemicals occur at concentrations even lower than the existing standards. The *Times* reported, "Studies indicate that drinking water contaminants are linked to millions of instances of illness within the United Stated each year." Half of all groundwater wells contain pesticide residues.

Phosphate fertilizers used in farming are a problem. Phosphate fertilizers are often contaminated with cadmium. The cadmium gets into the water supply and into the food, and people with high cadmium levels have high cancer rates. Another problem is nitrates, primarily from applying nitrogen fertilizers, which end up in the drinking water. In the body, they are metabolized into N-nitroso compounds that have been shown to cause tumors at multiple organ sites in every animal species tested. Humans with high nitrate exposure have higher cancer rates. Yet another problem is hexavalent chromium, which is used in industrial operations such as chrome plating and the manufacturing of plastics and dyes. It has been linked to liver and kidney damage in animals as well as to leukemia, stomach cancer, and other cancers. Hexavalent chromium has been found in the tap water of thirty-one out of thirty-five cities sampled. Of these cities, twenty-five had levels that exceeded safety standards. Sadly, even if your water is not contaminated with any of these substances, it may still be unsafe to drink. The problem is most tap water in the United States contains toxic chlorine and fluoride.

Chlorine

Chlorine is added to our drinking water to protect us from pathogens, but chlorine itself and the compounds it forms in the water damage your health. If you drink, bathe, shower, or swim in chlorinated water, you are inhaling and absorbing chlorine into your body, damaging genes and cells. Chlorine reacts with organic compounds in the water, forming cancer-causing organochlorine compounds, which are easily absorbed into our bodies and accumulate over time. The U.S. Council of Environmental Quality stated, "Cancer risk among people drinking chlorinated water is 93% higher than among those whose water does not contain chlorine." Hot water, used to shower, vaporizes the chlorine and other chlorinated chemicals in the water. These are both inhaled (damaging the lungs) and absorbed through the skin. Exposure to vaporized chlorine is 100 times more damaging than drinking chlorinated water. Higher levels of chlorine compounds have been found in the breast tissue of women with breast cancer.

Swimming in chlorinated water is especially dangerous. Chlorine penetrates the skin, gets into cells, damages DNA, and causes skin cancer. Beyond the chlorine itself, swimming pools and hot tubs often have high levels of toxic organochlorine compounds, which are absorbed through the skin or inhaled from the fumes near the surface of the pool or the tub. A study in the *European Respiratory Journal* found that young children who swim in chlorinated pools suffer permanent lung damage, increasing their lifelong risk of respiratory infections, allergies, and asthma. So-called saltwater pools are still chlorinated pools. Safe pool treatments are available and should be used.

Fluoride

Fluoridation is touted as one of the greatest public-health achievements of the twentieth century. In truth, it is one of the greatest public-health blunders of all time. Nearly 70 percent of the U.S. population drinks fluoridated tap water. Way back in 1975, Dean Burk, the former chief chemist at the National Cancer Institute, said that fluoridated water "causes more human cancer, and causes it faster, than any other chemical."

Fluoride is a general cellular poison. Yet many of us are now ingesting daily amounts that far exceed the government's inadequate safety standards. Hundreds of studies have found a connection between fluoride and cancer; cities that fluoridate have significantly more cancer deaths than cities that do not fluoridate. Fluoride causes cancer by inhibiting numerous essential enzymes and impairing oxygen respiration, which lowers energy production. Fluoride also inhibits production of thyroid hormones, causing an epidemic of thyroid disorders and hormonal imbalances. The pineal gland, located in the brain, produces melatonin. It plays a vital role in sleep and regulates puberty. Malfunction of this gland can lead to immune, digestive, respiratory, kidney, and blood circulation problems. The pineal accumulates more fluoride than any other soft tissue, and pineal fluoride levels are now high enough to cause problems, including girls reaching puberty at younger and younger ages.

Making matters worse, most fluoridated water contains arsenic. Fluorosilicic acid, the chemical most often used to fluoridate U.S. water systems, is a toxic waste by-product that comes from the pollution-scrubbing devices of the phosphate fertilizer industry. A contaminant commonly found in this product is arsenic. In 2001 the National Research Council warned, "Even very low concentrations of arsenic in drinking water appear to be associated with a higher incidence of cancer." Yet 90 percent of the arsenic in tap water comes from the fluoridation chemicals added to the water.

We get fluoride not only from our water but also from toothpaste and processed foods made with fluoridated water, including sodas, fruit juices, beer, and breakfast cereals. Many commercial fruit juices have been found to contain large amounts of fluoride. Crops watered with fluoridated water concentrate the fluoride and pass it on to you when you eat those foods. Tea leaves accumulate more fluoride than any other edible plant, and the fluoride content in tea has risen dramatically over the last couple of decades. Some teas contain alarming levels of fluoride due to the use of fluoride-containing fertilizers and pesticides. While the U.S. Environmental Protection Agency (EPA) allows only 4 parts per million (ppm) of fluoride in drinking water, it allows 900 ppm in powdered eggs, 125 ppm in wheat flour, and 70 ppm in processed foods. The average American is getting a daily toxic dose of fluoride that *far exceeds* the existing safety standards, which are already inadequate to protect us.

Fluoride levels found in tap water inhibit over 100 enzymes in the body, including critical DNA repair enzymes. Numerous studies have shown that fluoride can result in genetic damage at concentrations as low as 1 ppm, the amount commonly found in fluoridated drinking water. Fluoride bioaccumulates in our bodies, and the damage increases as the fluoride concentration goes up. Fluoride has been linked to dulled intellect in children, fragile bones, and bone cancer. One reason that older people have more cancer is that their ability to repair damaged DNA declines—as little as 1 ppm of fluoride can disrupt DNA repair enzymes by 50 percent.

Even 1 ppm of fluoride is capable of transforming normal cells into cancer cells. Research published in *Cell Biology and Toxicology* reported that a fluoride concentration of 1 ppm drives cancer, increasing tumor growth rates by 25 percent. Bone cancer rates in young men is six times higher in fluoridated communities.

Reduction of tooth decay is the justification for putting fluoride in tap water. However, numerous studies show that fluoride does nothing to protect teeth. In fact, cities that fluoridate often have higher cavity rates. Even worse, fluoride causes a type of poisoning called *dental fluorosis*, which manifests as a mottling and discoloration in the tooth enamel. Studies show that about one in four children have some degree of dental fluorosis. Fluorosis is a symptom of fluoride poisoning. In fact, x-rays of children with dental fluorosis often show bone abnormalities elsewhere in the body. This problem is called *skeletal fluorosis*, a disease that weakens bones in a manner similar to osteoporosis. According to the National Academy for the Advancement of Science, the minimum fluoride dosage that can cause skeletal fluorosis is 5 mg/day for twenty to forty years. Americans living in areas with fluoridated water average up to 6.6 mg/day. Not surprisingly, the United States has the world's highest hip fracture rate! Fluoride damages your bones and teeth by binding to minerals such as calcium and magnesium, creating deficiencies of these minerals at the cellular level. Robert Carton, Ph.D., a former EPA scientist, asserted in 1992, "Fluoridation is the greatest case of scientific fraud of this century."

Most people are unaware that the FDA has never approved adding fluoride to drinking water. We have been adding this toxin to our tap water for well over a half century, and yet the FDA still classifies fluoride as an "unapproved drug." The fact is that fluoride could never get FDA approval because it is toxic and ineffective. To avoid fluoride, use a reverse osmosis system to purify your drinking water, do not use fluoride toothpaste, and avoid processed foods.

Bottled Water

Is bottled water safe? If you can get bottled water from a high-quality source in glass bottles, the answer is yes. The quality of bottled water varies widely, and many brands have been found to be no better, and in some cases worse, than ordinary tap water, contaminated with chemicals and bacteria. In addition, toxins from the plastic bottles, such as carcinogenic BPA, can leach into the water. A high-quality reverse osmosis system removes chlorine, toxic chlorinated compounds, prescription drugs, arsenic, aluminum, fluoride, and other toxins from your drinking water. Put your home-filtered water in a glass bottle and carry it with you when you are away from home.

What's in Your Air?

Air pollution has been long recognized as causing ailments from allergies to cancer. Inhaling particles is known to disrupt the heart's beat-to-beat variations, and reduced heart rate variability has been associated with increased risk for mortality from all causes. An estimated 64,000 Americans die prematurely each year from heart and lung disease caused by particulate pollution. Even colds, flu, and asthma can result from the damage to immunity caused by breathing polluted air. However, you don't have to live downwind of a power plant or drive behind a truck to be poisoned by air pollution. While you may think of your home as your castle, it may be more like a toxic waste dump. Toxicity from indoor air pollution affects the health of virtually all Americans, producing a wide variety of symptoms, including anxiety, depression, fatigue, headaches, poor concentration, and poor mental acuity, as well as bodily aches and pains. When people complain of these symptoms, however, their physicians almost never suggest indoor pollutants as a probable (or even possible) cause. Home air filters are recommended.

Home Pollutants

Some of the most polluted air you can breathe is found right in your own home. The combination of indoor pollution and the fact that most Americans spend 90 percent of their time indoors creates a serious health challenge.

The multiple sources of indoor pollutants include polluted outside air with all its particles and chemicals coming into our homes as well as the pollution from building materials, furnishings, mattresses, gas appliances, furnaces, cleaning and consumer products, tobacco smoke, incense, deodorants, carpets, paint, household cleansers, copy machines, printers, electronic equipment, dry cleaning, newspapers, and magazines. Anything you can smell that is not natural is almost certainly toxic. The longer we breathe it, and the more concentrated it is, the more damage it inflicts, putting another burden on our already overstressed bodies. Indoor air is a health risk due to the combined effects of multiple toxic sources concentrated in a confined space.

Never use pesticides in or around the home. A 2006 study in the journal *Occupational and Environmental Medicine* found that the risk of developing leukemia was twice as likely in children whose mothers had used insecticides in the home before birth and long after birth. The use of insecticidal shampoos for head lice also doubled the risk of leukemia. Tobacco smoke, perfume, cosmetics, cleaning products, aerosol products, and all manner of scented products are toxic and should be avoided. Safe alternatives are available.

Paradichlorobenzene, found in mothballs and deodorizers, is another common indoor pollutant and also a carcinogen. Cedar chips are a more benign alternative to mothballs.

Cookware

Choosing what you eat is vital for your health, and choosing how you cook is also important. *Glass, Corningware, ceramics, and stainless are your best options.* Aluminum, iron, copper, and nonstick cookware are your worst options. Aluminum easily leeches into cooked foods, and the toxic effects of small amounts are cumulative and highly toxic. Iron and copper cookware both leach metals into the food that can accumulate to toxic levels. Nonstick coatings are made with perfluorocarbons (PFCs), which give off toxic fumes when heated. PFCs are also found in food wrappers, other consumer products, and seafood. They accumulate in the body and compromise the immune system.

Building Materials

Building materials themselves, such as plywood, particleboard, and paints, outgas formaldehyde and other chemicals into the air of your home. Formaldehyde causes serious damage to DNA, and the damage is cumulative as exposure continues. It is known to cause cancer. Houses and furniture made of particleboard greatly increase the amount of formaldehyde and other chemicals you breathe in your home. While the construction industry claims that safer particleboards have been available since the 1980s, they too outgas toxic chemicals and are still not safe.

Carpets

Carpets made of synthetic fibers outgas copious amounts of toxic chemicals, some of them for decades. New carpets are especially toxic. Synthetic-fiber carpets can contain as many as 200 toxic chemicals that outgas from the fibers, dyes, adhesives, backing, fire retardants, fungicides, antistatic and stain-resistant treatments, and padding. Researchers at Anderson Labs measured the effects of carpet toxicity on 110 families and found that 82 percent developed diverse health problems within three months of installation, including irregular heartbeat, fatigue, rashes, memory loss, muscle pain, blurred vision, and tremors. Mice exposed to fumes from new carpets died in a matter of hours, while carpets up to twelve years old caused neurological problems. Install only natural-fiber carpets, tile, stone, or hardwood floors with natural-fiber area rugs.

Appliances

Dangerous gases and particles are generated by household appliances such as gas stoves, water heaters, furnaces, space heaters, and fireplaces, which can release toxins such as nitrogen dioxide, carbon monoxide, methane, and other gases, along with fine particles, into the indoor air. Furnaces and gas water heaters should be kept outside the living space, such as in a shed or unattached garage. If this is not possible, consider switching to an electric water heater. Gas stoves should be used only with good ventilation; an electric stove is preferable. Use fireplaces sparingly, and never use artificial logs, as they put a heavy hydrocarbon load into the living space.

Hot water used in dishwashers, clothes washers, bathtubs, and showers vaporizes the chlorine and other chemicals in the tap water, as well as the bleaches or detergents being used. Exposure by breathing these chemicals exceeds exposure from drinking the water because the inhaled gases go directly into the bloodstream. In fact, about two-thirds of our exposure to chlorine results from inhalation of steam and skin absorption when showering. Good ventilation is essential. Best is to filter the chlorine out of your shower water. Shower filters and whole-house filters are readily available.

Cars

New cars are particularly dangerous. The chemicals contained in a new car's plastics, adhesives, and seating materials pollute the interior air of the car with known endocrine disrupters and carcinogens. One class of these chemicals is called *phthalates*, which disrupt normal hormone function by mimicking estrogen. Phthalates—also found in plastic bottles, food packaging, hoses, shower curtains, vinyl wall coverings, toys, cosmetics, hair conditioners, and fragrances—cause sexual development abnormalities in children and contribute to cancer. During the first several months, leave a new car parked in the hot sun with the windows up to bake out the toxins. Air it out regularly, and be sure to air it out before you drive and keep it well ventilated while driving.

Attached garages can be another problem. Exhaust fumes as well as hydrocarbon vapors coming from the engine can enter the living space. Whenever possible, leave the garage door open to ventilate that space, especially after returning from a trip where the engine and oil are hot.

Smoking

Smoking is a worldwide epidemic and a self-destructive addiction that can be a major source of indoor pollution. Cigarette smoke contains over 4,000 different chemicals, most of which are toxic, plus airborne particulates. These toxins make you sick, accelerate aging, depress immunity, and cause cancer. The tars cause obstructive lung disease, and the nicotine increases heart rate and blood pressure. Smoking also increases the stickiness of blood platelets, which increases the risk of blood clots.

Airborne Particles

The average American breathes in about two heaping tablespoons of airborne particles each day. The smallest of these particles are capable of lodging deep in the lungs where they remain and cause serious problems. In 2004, Canadian researchers reported in the journal *Science* that fine airborne particles can cause genetic mutations that are passed on to future generations. Such damage is fundamental in the development of cancer. Most of these fine particles emanate from industrial plants, power plants, incinerators, and diesel-burning vehicles. A study of Los Angeles air concluded that 71 percent of the cancer risk from air contaminants came from diesel emissions. Fireplaces and woodstoves are another source of airborne particles.

All Americans need to reduce their toxic load and to be aware of the health risks that air pollution poses. To protect ourselves, we must begin with our personal environment and stop introducing pollutants. Be aware of the problems with carpets, paints, cleaning materials, deodorizers, mattresses, gas appliances, fragrances, dry cleaning chemicals, fireplaces, and so forth.

Work to reduce the amount of pollutants you introduce into your environment. Toward this end, use filters: shower, drinking water, and air filters. You can prevent genetic damage from fine-particle exposure by filtering the air with a HEPA filter. Due to the unprecedented levels of air pollution to which we are now exposed, air filters have become a virtual necessity, especially if you live in an urban environment or are near a heavily traveled highway with diesel emissions. High-quality water and air filters are available through *www.beyondhealth.com.*

Other Sources of Toxins

Look in your bathrooms. Likely there are enough toxic chemicals there to make anybody sick. The toxic products include toilet bowl cleaners, hair spray, and deodorizers, in addition to the toxic chlorinated water coming out of the tap. Toilet deodorizers are made from paradichlorobenzene, the same carcinogenic chemical found in mothballs. All of these products can be replaced with safer, simpler, yet effective items available in health food stores.

Your laundry room is another toxic site. Detergents, bleach, spot removers, and fabric softeners all contain chemicals that are toxic to you and to the environment. Detergents can be replaced with soap-based products, while bleach can be replaced with safer oxygen bleaches such as sodium percarbonate and hydrogen peroxide. Purchase unscented products.

Household furniture often is made with toxic synthetic materials (polyester, polyurethane, polystyrene, and polyvinyl chloride), which outgas toxins and present significant health risks. Today, furniture is commonly made of particleboard and then covered with a wood or plastic veneer. Alarmingly, most children's furniture is made with toxic particleboard. Buy furniture made from natural materials, such as solid wood or metal. Another less expensive option is used furniture made of natural materials. The typical crib mattress outgases up to thirty different volatile organic compounds. Infants are particularly vulnerable to toxins, and most of them spend much of their first year in a crib where they are being poisoned with toxic chemicals that can have a lifelong effect on their health. *Everyone* should be sleeping on nontoxic mattresses.

Even the clothes you wear can be toxic. Have you ever gone into a clothing store and noticed the chemical-laden atmosphere? That unhealthy atmosphere results from the fact that most clothes today contain or are made of toxic synthetic fibers (such as nylon, polyester, acrylics, and spandex). The chemicals outgassing from these fibers as well as their dyes, formaldehyde finishes (permanent press), and mothproofing pesticides will affect you as you wear them and contribute to toxic air in your home. Dry cleaning brings toxins into your household. Clothes that have been dry-cleaned should always be aired out thoroughly before they are put into a closet or worn. Many people are quite sensitive to residues from laundry detergents and fabric softeners. Have you ever walked down the detergent aisle at the grocery store and had your eyes, nose, or throat feel irritated? Toxins in those boxes are outgassing. When washing your clothes, use environmentally friendly and unscented laundry products such as the Seventh Generation brand. Do not use scented fabric softeners. These products might make your clothes smell "clean and fresh," but that smell is toxic. Buy clothes made of natural materials such as wool and cotton, and use natural cleaning products.

Keep your home or office well ventilated. To save on energy costs, modern homes and office buildings are built a lot tighter than older construction. While reducing energy waste is good, reducing air circulation allows pollutants to accumulate to higher concentrations. This is why high-quality air filters (that filter out both airborne particles and chemicals) can be helpful. Use them in rooms where you spend a great lot time, such as your office or bedroom.

Obvious though it sounds, the most important thing you can do to keep your indoor air clean is to stop introducing pollutants in the first place. Before purchasing something new, consider if that product might contribute to your indoor pollution. As mentioned earlier, after buying

something, give it a chance to outgas before putting it in your living environment. Do not use products that have powerful chemical odors, such as mothballs or air fresheners. Whenever possible, use heat or direct sunshine to help accelerate the outgassing process.

Prescription Drugs

A major source of avoidable toxins is prescription drugs. Drugs are extremely toxic and almost always unnecessary. William Osler, M.D., once said, "The person who takes medicine must recover twice. Once from the disease and once from the medicine." When we finally get sick from our poor nutrition and toxic overload, most of us go to conventional physicians. Not knowing any better, physicians prescribe drugs, which increase your toxic load, make you even sicker, and perhaps even kill you. Prescription drugs are so toxic that millions of people are hospitalized each year due to adverse reactions to them, and an estimated several hundred thousand are killed. In fact, properly prescribed drugs are the third-leading cause of death in the United States. Just think, we could eliminate the third-leading cause of death by simply outlawing prescription drugs. Not only could we save hundreds of thousands of lives each year, but we would also reduce healthcare costs by hundreds of billions of dollars. Best of all, overall health and quality of life would actually improve.

There might be justification for using drugs if they served a useful purpose, but drugs do nothing to cure disease and many are little better than placebos. The top-selling drugs in the world are cholesterol-lowering drugs. Yet here is what a 1996 study in the *Journal of the American Medical Association* had to say about this class of drugs: "All members of the two most popular classes of lipid-lowering drugs (the fibrates and the statins) cause cancer in rodents, in some cases at levels of animal exposure close to those prescribed to humans."

By the time you are on more than a couple of prescription drugs, no one in the world knows what is going on in your body; every cell is being poisoned. The healthiest person alive will get sick if they take prescription drugs, but sick people are already compromised and have less ability to metabolize these chemicals and protect themselves from their toxic effects.

Sales of prescription drugs are soaring. Americans represent 4 percent of the world's population, yet they take 50 percent of all the prescription drugs produced in the world. Since drugs cause disease, this helps to explain why the health of the American people is so poor when compared to other nations. Half of all Americans now take at least one prescription drug. One out of four children takes at least one prescription drug. Many of our elderly take a dozen or more drugs per day. It's no wonder they are losing their minds, unstable on their feet, feeling fatigued, and their health is in a downward spiral. These drugs put a huge toxic load on us and on the environment. Alarming amounts of prescription drugs are now showing up in our water supply, poisoning fish and animals that depend on that water, not to mention poisoning young children who drink that water. Fortunately, drugs are unnecessary. It is difficult to think of a drug for which there is not a safer, less expensive, and more effective alternative.

Personal Care Products

Most people assume that the chemicals in their personal care and other household consumer products have been tested for safety and proved to be safe. Not so! Almost all personal care products—toothpaste, antibacterial soaps, shaving cream, aftershave, nail polish, deodorant products, skin lotions, hair sprays, hair dyes, fragrances, shampoos, and conditioners—contain toxic chemicals that add to your toxic overload. At least one-third of the chemicals used to make these products have already been identified as contributing to cancer or other serious health problems. In addition, these chemicals acting in combination are much more toxic than any one of them acting alone. Some of these chemicals are endocrine disrupters that affect hormonal balance, leading to numerous problems, including mood swings and cancer. Suntan lotions contain at least half a dozen chemicals that have been identified as carcinogens or endocrine disrupters. Most people don't even conceive that products as common as toothpaste or shampoo are significant sources of dangerous toxins that are making them sick.

Especially important are products you put in your mouth or on your skin. Toxins you swallow are subjected to enzymes in your stomach, and then pass through the liver, so they are broken down before they reach the rest of your body. When toxins are absorbed through the mucous membranes in the mouth or through the skin, they can enter the bloodstream and your tissues without the above protective effects. The same toxin can be 100 times more toxic when absorbed through the skin or mucous membranes than when swallowed, so be especially cautious when using products like mouthwash, toothpaste, shampoo, and skin lotions.

Most skin-care products, even the most expensive brands, contain a variety of toxic chemicals that damage your health, damage your skin, and add years to your appearance. Studies show that these ingredients damage sublayers of skin, causing you to look older and promoting skin irritation and redness, more wrinkles, more age spots, and sagging skin. Many products contain petroleum-derived mineral oil, paraffin, and petrolatum that are suspected carcinogens and hormone disrupters. Parabens are common preservatives used in personal care products, and they, too, are hormone disrupters and suspected carcinogens. Sodium laurel or lauryl sulfate is included in over 90 percent of personal care products.

They break down the skin's moisture barrier, easily allowing other chemicals to penetrate the skin, and they combine with other chemicals, forming powerful carcinogens. Acrylamide, linked to tumors in laboratory research, is found in many hand and face creams. Dioxane is a powerful carcinogen, and it can be found as a contaminant in common ingredients such as PEG, polysorbates, laureth, and ethoxylated alcohols. Other toxins include phenol (carbolic acid) and propylene glycol.

Toothpaste is something most people use daily without realizing it is a dangerous source of toxins. Read the warning label on the box: if you swallow more than a little, you should seek medical assistance. Toothpaste contains a deadly mixture of toxins, such as fluoride; artificial colors, flavors, and sweeteners; and synthetic detergents like sodium lauryl sulfate. All of these can pass through the mucous membranes and bioaccumulate in the body, leading to toxic overload and disease. The mucous membranes in your mouth are very permeable, so if you expose yourself to toxic toothpaste daily, you are bioaccumulating a lot of toxins. Like other personal care products, there are safe brands of toothpaste, such as the Weleda brand.

Shampoo is another toxin-loaded product that many use daily. Shampoos contain synthetic detergents such as sodium lauryl sulfate (SLS). SLS itself is neurotoxic, unbalances hormones, and disrupts normal cell chemistry. In addition, SLS is frequently contaminated with 1,4-dioxane, which is toxic to the liver, kidneys, and brain, but also is listed as a probable human carcinogen. Dioxane has even been found in baby shampoo. These toxins pass through the skin and bioaccumulate in tissues to levels that cause serious cellular malfunction and disease.

Shampoos also contain preservatives such as parabens. The EPA has linked parabens to hormonal, neurological, metabolic, and developmental disorders, and to cancer. Researchers have found parabens in every sample of breast cancer tissue. Propylene glycol is another problem. Found in numerous shampoo and skincare products, it is a skin irritant known to cause liver and kidney damage. Shampoos also contain artificial colors, which have been shown to be carcinogenic when applied to the skin. Here is what the Center for Science in the Public Interest had to say regarding artificial colors: "The three most widely used dyes, Red 40, Yellow 5, and Yellow 6, are contaminated with known carcinogens. . . . Another dye, Red 3, has been acknowledged for years by the Food and Drug Administration to be a carcinogen, yet is still in the food supply." Some safe shampoos, such as the Aubrey Organics brand, don't have these harmful ingredients.

A study by the University of Southern California published in the *International Journal of Cancer* revealed that monthly use of permanent hair dye when used for twelve months doubled the risk of bladder cancer. The risk tripled after fifteen years of use. Temporary or semipermanent dyes did not have the same risks, according to the researchers.

The largest category of cosmetic and personal care products is perfumes, colognes, and fragrances. Even high-end perfumes are made with cocktails of dangerous and untested chemicals that can produce problems from allergies to hormone disruption and cancer. According to the Environmental Working Group, most perfumes contain an average of ten known allergens that can trigger reactions from asthma to headaches to contact dermatitis, and an average of four chemicals known to disrupt the hormonal (endocrine) system. These endocrine disrupters have been linked to reproductive defects in male infants, sperm damage in men, and more recently, hyperactivity in children.

Fragrances are extensively used in a wide range of household cleaning products. The industry uses more than 5,000 different chemicals to make synthetic fragrances. Among them are hormone-disrupting chemicals like phthalates and toxic solvents like xylene and toluene. Toluene is found in most synthetic fragrances, and chronic exposure can cause anemia, low blood cell count, liver or kidney damage, and damage to a fetus. These ingredients are not regulated, and they do not need to be listed on the label. Some of these chemicals are known to cause allergies and cancer and do reproductive and hormonal damage. If you must use a fragrance, use a natural essential oil derived from flowers and natural herbs; natural oils are available at health food and specialty stores.

Fortunately, safe personal care products—such as toothpastes, shampoos, skin creams, and deodorants—are available. All you have to do is choose them. This will lower your toxic load, put less of a burden on your overworked immune system and help you to better prevent and reverse disease.

The Importance of Hormone-Disrupting Chemicals

No one fully understands the impact of the hormone-disrupting chemicals in our environment, but the more we learn, the more catastrophic they appear to be. Endocrine-disrupting chemicals (EDCs), found in numerous household and industrial products, interfere with the action of hormones in the body, throwing the body out of regulation and causing disease. We are only starting to understand the ramifications of these chemicals on our health, and the indications are that they are having serious effects, causing asthma, cancer, cognitive decline, diabetes, infertility, and even obesity.

A 2012 update to a World Health Organization report on endocrine-disrupting chemicals found that babies exposed to EDCs in the womb are at higher risk for developing behavioral and learning disorders. The report also cited a higher incidence of adrenal, bone, thyroid, and metabolic disorders from EDC exposure. Cancer of the endocrine glands, such as the breast, prostate, and thyroid glands, is now epidemic.

Unfortunately, EDCs are now everywhere in our environment and are almost impossible to avoid. There are about 800 different types of EDCs, and they include parabens, phthalates, insecticides, and poly-brominated flame retardants. The task is to avoid as many as possible. Bisphenol-A (BPA) is an important EDC. In 2009, more than 2 million tons of BPA were produced worldwide. This ended up in common consumer products such as the paper used in purchase receipts, the linings of food and beverage cans, and plastic water and beverage bottles. Animal studies show a direct correlation between BPA and breast cancer. Other sources of EDCs include air fresheners, cosmetics, hair dyes, household cleaning products, synthetic fragrances and perfumes, pharmaceuticals, toys, and even sunscreens.

Handle cash register receipts carefully and wash your hands after touching them. Do not drink or eat products packaged in cans. Do not use plastic water bottles. Limit use of canned foods and beverages. Use only safe, natural brands of cosmetics, personal care products, perfumes, and cleaning products.

Mothers

Mothers must exercise special care to detoxify before becoming pregnant because they risk poisoning their children. Toxins in the mother's blood are transferred to the fetus, which is causing an epidemic of disease in our children. After accidents, cancer is the leading cause of death for children. Neurodevelopmental disorders in children have increased dramatically over the last few decades, and one in six U.S. children now has such a disorder. One cause is mercury accumulation in the mother. A 2008 study in *Environmental Health Perspectives* found that one in three

U.S. infants have a cord blood mercury level that exceeds EPA safety standards, and that the cord blood mercury level was over twice the level found in the blood of the mothers. Furthermore, testing of these children at thirty-six and forty-eight months found that the children with the most mercury had the lowest performance, verbal, and IQ scores. When aluminum and lead are also present, a common occurrence, mercury becomes 100 times more toxic.

In addition to the problems with cord blood, mother's milk in U.S. women is highly contaminated. Pesticides, flame retardants, and other toxic chemicals are found in the milk. Exposure to these toxins needs to be reduced before pregnancy.

Support Your Detoxification System

Not allowing toxins to enter your body is the first step in winning the battle against toxic overload. The next step is to support your detoxification systems. We are not only exposed to external toxins from our foods, the air, and water, but our cells generate a huge amount of toxins every day in the form of waste products from normal metabolism. Fortunately, we have exquisitely designed detoxification systems to dispose of these chemicals safely. Unfortunately, we are overloading these systems. Overloading is bad enough, but our poor diets lack the nutrients these detox systems need to do their jobs.

The liver is our major detoxification organ. Anything you can do to ease its toxic burden will make the liver's job easier and benefit your health. Enzymes produced by the liver deactivate and eliminate toxins. If these enzymes are deactivated by environmental toxins such as lead and mercury—or never manufactured in the first place because of nutrient deficiency—toxin-caused diseases are certain to result. Liver-enzyme detoxification has two phases. In Phase I, the liver produces enzymes that take harmful toxins such as alcohol, pesticides, herbicides, and prescription drugs, and oxidizes them in preparation for removal from the body. This process creates potentially harmful free radicals that must be neutralized by antioxidants. In Phase II, more enzymes are used to combine the oxidized chemicals from Phase I with other molecules so that they can be excreted harmlessly in the bile or urine. These elegant systems do a fabulous job, but they depend on a constant supply of critical nutrients to function properly. In both phases, the food we eat or supplements we take must supply the raw materials needed to produce all of these enzymes, antioxidants, and other chemicals. Unfortunately, the average diet does not supply what we need, so we get sick.

Support your liver's Phase I detoxification process with antioxidant nutrients. Vitamins A, C, and E along with coenzyme Q10, bioflavonoids, carotenoids, copper, manganese, selenium, and zinc are needed. Some of these nutrients neutralize free radicals directly; others support enzymes that neutralize them. Red, yellow, and green vegetables are loaded with these antioxidant nutrients. You can assist Phase II detoxification with cruciferous vegetables such as cabbage, broccoli, cauliflower, green onions, kale, and Brussels sprouts. These vegetables enable the liver to eliminate powerful carcinogens, helping to protect against cancer. These dietary suggestions, combined with high-quality supplements, will keep your liver's toxic defenses at peak function. Juicing vegetables every day helps by making more of these precious chemicals biologically available.

Reducing Stored Toxins

Americans are probably the most toxic creatures on the planet, and the amount of stored toxins in our cells and tissues has reached crisis levels. Unless you are taking active measures to reduce your toxic load, then each day you are adding to them. As you grow older, your toxic load will reach catastrophic levels and make you sick. We cannot afford to continue adding to our toxic load; we need to be subtracting from it. Different approaches to reducing stored toxins include the following.

Saunas

Avoiding toxins is essential, but getting rid of stored toxins is the other half of the equation. One powerful solution is a sauna. Heat causes cells to release toxins; cultures around the world for millennia have used hyperthermic (sweat) treatments. The ancient Egyptians, Greeks, and Romans—and even American Indians—used such treatments. Hyperthermic practices are known to reduce levels of oil-soluble toxins, such as pesticides and PCBs. Saunas melt the fat layer in the skin, allowing the oil to ooze out of the oil glands along with its cargo of accumulated fat-soluble toxins. In addition, water-soluble toxins are lost in the sweat, carrying out heavy metals like lead and mercury. Over time, it is possible to reduce one's toxic load substantially as well as keep it low.

With almost every American in toxic overload, using a sauna on a regular basis has become a necessity for achieving and maintaining good health. Sherry Rogers, M.D., an internationally known expert in environmental medicine and author of *Tired or Toxic*, maintains that saunas have become "a household necessity." According to Dr. Rogers,

> *A sauna used to be thought of as a luxury. But studies now confirm that diet and environmental chemicals cause 95 percent of cancers. Furthermore, as the first generation of man exposed to an unprecedented plethora of daily chemicals, we have learned that stored chemicals can mimic any disease. "Incurable" chronic diseases that were thought to have no known cause often disappear when toxic chemicals are gone.*

Over the last century, our environment has become a sea of petroleum-based, oil-soluble toxins. Never before exposed to these chemicals, nature did not design a way for us to get rid of them. The average person is now bioaccumulating between 300 and 500 man-made chemicals. Styrene (found in plastic drinking cups and food packaging) is now found in 100 percent of human tissue in America. PCBs, dioxins, para-dichlorobenzene (found in mothballs and deodorizers), sodium lauryl sulfate (found in soap, shampoo, and toothpaste), triclosan (found in antibacterial soap and underarm deodorants), and many others are all bioaccumulating in our tissues. Many of these chemicals are known carcinogens. Many are hormone disrupters, which helps to explain why so many of us have hormonal abnormalities, why children are entering puberty at younger and younger ages, and why we have so many hormone-driven cancers such as breast and prostate cancers. In addition to reducing the environmental chemical burden, sweating in a sauna helps to manage pH and maintain the acid/alkaline balance by getting rid of the lactic acid produced by metabolizing sugars.

After completing a sauna, it is essential to wash off immediately with a good castile soap, which rinses the toxins off so that they don't reabsorb into the skin. Regular use of a conventional sauna is effective, but far infrared saunas are an even more efficient and effective way to remove stored toxins.

If you use a commercial sauna at a gym or health club, lie prone on the lowest bench. This will expose your body to a manageable temperature, allowing you to spend more time. Start slowly and gradually work your way up to an hour or more. Saunas played a critical role in reducing my toxic overload and restoring my health when I was at death's door. Even now, I still sauna twice a week for sixty to ninety minutes to keep my toxic load down. You can use your sauna time to do other healthy things such as meditation. I even use it to return phone calls.

Many people cannot tolerate conventional saunas due to the excessively hot air. Even under these harsh conditions, the heat penetration from conventional saunas is superficial, penetrating only a few millimeters. Infrared saunas are a completely different experience. The infrared heats you rather than the air, so the air temperature is kept at a comfortable and controllable level—105 to 115 degrees versus 130 to 180 degrees in a conventional sauna. Meanwhile, the penetration is over one and a half inches deep, which is desirable for healing tissue and releasing toxins.

If you have not used a sauna before, it may take some getting used to. Work your way up in time slowly, and if you ever feel faint, dizzy, or sick, get out. Over time, you will get used to it. Also, keep hydrated when using a sauna. A combination of daily exercise, nutritional supplements, and a regular sauna has a powerfully beneficial effect on health.

Fasting

Fasting is the complete abstinence from all substances except pure water, in a restful environment. Juice fasting, a popular variation, is abstinence from all food and drink except water and fresh vegetable juices. People have been fasting for thousands of years, both for spiritual and health purposes. It is an integral part of many religions, including Islam, Judaism, and Christianity. Fasting is a powerful way of detoxifying and is known to have a beneficial effect on health. As far back as 400 BC, Hippocrates prescribed total abstinence from food while a disease was on the increase. Ancient priests provided sanctuaries where people could go to fast.

Fasting promotes detoxification. The body normally eliminates or neutralizes toxins through the colon, liver, kidneys, lungs, lymph nodes, and skin. Fasting helps this process because when you are no longer eating food, the body turns to its fat reserves for energy. As the fat reserves are burned, they release their stored toxins, which are then eliminated through the usual organs mentioned above.

Fasting also triggers the healing process. The body uses lots of energy to digest food. During a fast, energy is diverted away from the digestive system toward the metabolism and immune system. When fasting, the body naturally searches for dead cells, damaged tissues, fatty deposits, tumors, and abscesses, tearing them down so that they can be burned for fuel or expelled as waste. During fasting, the body also rebuilds damaged tissues. Fasting allows the digestive system to repair itself, restoring good digestion and elimination. The elimination of problem areas restores the immune system and metabolic functionality to an optimum state, rejuvenating the body and giving it a more youthful tone. The benefits of fasting can have lasting effects on your physical, mental, and emotional health.

Another benefit of fasting is weight loss. Intermittent fasting is an excellent weight-loss strategy. At the same time, it reduces inflammation, improves blood sugar levels, and reduces cholesterol. In this way, it can help to prevent and control diabetes.

During a simple water fast, all you consume is water. Make sure to consume plenty of pure water to help flush toxins through your system as your body uses its energy to release them. Avoid water straight from the faucet. Distilled water from a pure, natural source or reverse osmosis water is the best for cleansing. Drink at least two liters per day. I stir buffered vitamin C powder into water throughout the day, which provides extra antioxidant power to protect against free radicals while helping the body to detoxify. Organic lemon juice in pure water can also be helpful in the cleansing process, as lemon supports the liver. If you desire to make fasting a habit, an excellent book to teach you about fasting is *Toxic Relief* by Dr. Don Colbert, M.D.

In many situations, fasting is the only known solution. Fasting dissolves tumors. As the body searches for energy sources, abnormal growths such as tumors are more likely to be self-digested by the body's natural enzymes. To overcome a severe disease like cancer, it is usually necessary to continue through a series of fasts to remove all the tumor tissue. Many people have overcome cancer with fasting. Fasting has also been beneficial for arthritis, asthma, high blood pressure, high cholesterol, lupus, chronic fatigue, colitis, Crohn's disease, diverticulitis, spastic colon, irritable bowel, cases of paralysis, neuritis, neuralgia, neuroses, insomnia, addictions, mental illness, and other health problems.

Aside from the usual nightly fasts while we are sleeping, giving our body more extended times of fasting is a healthy new habit to cultivate. Whether you begin by just fasting one meal a day, two meals a day, or one day a week, your body will have extra time to cleanse and detoxify. In fact, fasting is the one practice proven to extend life—fasting two days a week can double the life span of test animals.

Making a habit of fasting one day a week is not difficult, and it gives your body fifty-two days a year (a total of over seven weeks) to rest and detoxify. Some people prefer to fast three or four days in a row each month. I normally fast one day per week, taking only water with buffered vitamin C dissolved in it. Once a year, I fast for seven to ten days in a row and feel fabulous afterward. In fact, a ten-day fast helped to turn around my own serious health problems after I almost died from liver failure caused by a toxic prescription drug.

Longer fasts are preferable to short ones because once the body is in the fasting state, systemic cleansing is able to reach deeper into the body tissues. For this reason, most of the recoveries from serious illnesses have taken place with longer fasts, where a medically supervised fast of thirty to forty days may be required. There are excellent clinics where you can go for such fasts, and often all or part of the cost is reimbursable through medical insurance policies. Regular fasting is one habit that will reward you with benefits, including weight reduction and a longer life.

Conclusion

Toxins are a major cause of our epidemic of chronic disease. Reducing your toxic overload is essential for preventing or reversing disease. Toxins harm you in many ways. They reduce cell oxygenation, damage DNA, interrupt critical communications, give inappropriate instructions to genes, and shut down essential metabolic machinery. The resulting biochemical chaos interferes with the body's ability to self-repair, self-regulate, and keep you healthy.

As you've just found out, toxins are everywhere. Just because you can't see it, taste it, or smell it doesn't mean it can't harm you. If you can smell it and it's a man-made smell—such as a new car or new carpet smell—it's toxic, so limit your exposure as best you can.

How do you begin? There are simple things anyone can do. Get the processed foods out of your life along with their artificial colors, flavor enhancers, preservatives, and other chemical additives. Filter your drinking water; a reverse osmosis system is best. Filter your shower water, consider a whole-house filtration system. Avoid chlorinated pools and spas. Don't take drugs of any kind. Use safe personal care and household-cleaning products. Don't use artificial sweeteners. Support your liver's detoxification processes and take regular saunas. Once you start making these choices, they will become part of your daily living, and you will soon be making them without even thinking about it.

Do not microwave food; even healthy foods come out altered in ways that are toxic. As much as possible, eat only fresh organic foods. Banish all artificial sweeteners from your life! Get rid of toxic household clean-ing products and replace them with safe, ecologically sound alternatives. Upgrade your personal care products as well. Think twice about putting anything on your skin that you wouldn't eat, because much of what you apply topically does in fact get into your body. Avoid toothpastes with fluoride and antiperspirants with aluminum compounds.

Remember that prescription medications do not cure disease. They cause disease. Always look for alternatives to taking drugs as a long-term strategy. Especially avoid vaccinations and antibiotics whenever possible. They do permanent damage to your health. The much better approach is to strengthen your immune system so that you don't have to worry about infections.

Avoid charbroiling and other cooking methods that blacken foods. Support your liver's detoxification processes by supplementing with vita-mins A, C, and E; coenzyme Q10; selenium; manganese; copper; and zinc, and be sure to eat plenty of cruciferous vegetables like cabbage, broccoli, cauliflower, green onions, kale, and Brussels sprouts.

Avoid medical x-rays and opt out of the airport scanners. Avoid chlo-rinated pools and spas—use purification systems that do not depend on chlorine. Get your mercury amalgam fillings removed—but only by a dentist specially trained in safe mercury removal. Take long and frequent saunas to eliminate fat-soluble toxins.

Unless you stop putting toxins into your body and then get rid of stored toxins, your toxic load will continue to build up and cause cel-lular malfunction and disease. For women who wish to have children, addressing toxic overload is especially important to protect the children from birth defects, neurological damage, and cancer.

YOUR MAINTENANCE LIST
FOR THE TOXIN PATHWAY:

Energy Production

Avoid heavy metals, like lead and mercury that disable enzymes needed for energy production.

Avoid fluoride. It inhibits energy-producing enzymes.

Eliminating toxins through saunas and fasting gives you more energy.

Inflammation

Reduce toxins to reduce inflammation.

Take saunas to reduce inflammation.

Fast to reduce inflammation.

Acid/Alkaline Balance

Take saunas to maintain pH balance by getting rid of lactic acid through sweating.

Digestive Health

Avoid heavy metals. They shut down digestive enzymes.

Avoid fluoride. It accumulates in the pineal gland, leading to digestive problems.

Don't compromise your liver's ability to metabolize food with an overload of toxins.

Use periodic fasting to allow the digestive system to repair itself.

Hormonal Balance

Avoid heavy metal toxins. They disable enzymes needed for producing hormones.

Avoid endocrine-disrupting chemicals. They give false signals to cells and genes.

Avoid tap water, because it contains prescription drug residues, including sex hormones.

Avoid commercial meat, dairy, and farmed fish. They are contaminated with hormones.

Avoid fluoridated water. It inhibits the production of thyroid hormones.

Choose personal care products carefully. Many contain endocrine disrupters.

Take saunas and fast to release hormone disrupters stored in fat cells.

Platelet Stickiness

Avoid smoking. It increases the stickiness of blood platelets.

Fat Storage

Do periodic fasts to deplete fat reserves.

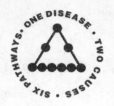

EIGHT

Using Your Mind to Heal

*The first place we must win the victory is
in our own minds. . . . If you don't think your
body can be healed, it never will be.*

—Joel Osteen, *Your Best Life Now*

*The simple truth is, happy people generally don't get sick.
One's attitude toward oneself is the single most
important factor in healing or staying well.*

—Bernie Siegel, M.D.,
Love, Medicine, and Miracles

*Wherever you go, no matter what the weather,
always bring your own sunshine.*

—Anthony J. D'Angelo

The Power of Mind over Matter

T   *he power of the mind to heal or make you sick is almost limitless.* Your nervous system is the master computer that checks, balances, and controls all the other systems in your body. Every thought and emotion trigger the release of chemical messengers throughout the body. In other words, there is no such thing as "just a thought." *Every thought has a physical consequence, for better or for worse.* This Mental Pathway chapter will help you think in new ways about your thoughts.

One of the greatest mysteries in medicine is the spontaneous remission of supposedly incurable chronic diseases. Thoughts and emotions are among the most important factors contributing to all disease. This is why a change in your thinking or belief can actually change how your genes express—same genes, different results. That's powerful! What you think can mean the difference between having or not having disease. Just as you are what you eat, you are what you think. Just as you can choose what you eat, you can choose what you think. *If you are sick and want to get well, you must change both what you eat and what you think.*

The U.S. Centers for Disease Control and Prevention (CDC) has stated that 85 percent of all diseases have an emotional component. Feelings of anger, apathy, gloom, and resentment weaken the immune system and damage health. Positive thoughts of love, compassion, joy, and humor support good health. Your mind is the biggest pharmacy on the planet, and it matters a great deal how you use it. Modern research has shown that your thoughts, emotions, and beliefs trigger the brain to produce a large variety of biologically active chemicals. The activities of the mind affect every body function, directly affecting how your cells operate.

In the mid-1970s, Hans Selye, M.D., was the first to demonstrate that animals subjected to stress experienced depressed immunity, elevated blood pressure, elevated triglycerides, and stomach ulcers. Since then, thousands of human studies have shown a direct link between mental state and disease, including cancer. How you handle stress makes a big difference. The same stressful event will make one person sick and have no effect on another, depending on how each chooses to react to that event. In essence, you can think your way into and out of disease. The power of the mind to heal is absolutely enormous.

As a result of decades of research, we now know that human intention can directly influence cell chemistry. This knowledge helps to explain the placebo effect, spontaneous remission, and the value of faith and prayer in human health. Thousands of years of human history tell us that the mind has a major impact on the body. In fact, research studies indicate that when conventional medicine's drugs and surgery work, it is because of the belief that the patient has in their efficacy. Belief is so powerful that it can even overcome the damage done by drugs and surgery and still make you well. It would be better and less expensive to harness that belief and skip the drugs and surgery.

Lack of purpose, low self-esteem, helplessness, hopelessness, anxiety, loneliness, depression, extreme mental or physical stress, or stressful life events, such as loss of a loved one, have all been proven to be immune-suppressing and cancer-promoting factors. For example, depression has been found to double the risk of cancer. A National Cancer Institute study found that the survival of cancer patients could be predicted with complete accuracy just based on their mental attitude and their will to live. People who beat the odds have a fighting spirit, live fully in the moment, and anticipate the future.

Our genes run the show, but the same gene produces different results based on the instructions we give to it. A strong and unambiguous intention to heal gives your genes the instructions they need to produce health-enhancing chemicals. Positive thoughts cause the creation of happy brain chemicals such as enkephalins and endorphins. Both these chemicals increase the production of immune T cells. But in addition to producing more T cells, positive thoughts cause something magical to happen: the vigor with which the T cells attack cancer cells and infections is also increased. Positive thoughts increase immunity. Negative thoughts have the opposite effect.

It is a scientific fact that your thoughts directly influence your physical being, so why not make that work for you instead of against you? Quantum physicists tell us we are made of frozen light, like an ice cube is made of frozen water. See yourself as what you really are—a being of light. That light is perfect, and so are you. See yourself as a body of perfect light. Constantly remind yourself of this fact. You are a perfect being; your perfection is the truth—not disease. The Bible says, "The truth will set you free." Live in the truth, meditate on the truth, and incorporate it into your being. You will be astonished at the power you unleash.

The Effects of Stress

Stress affects all of your maintenance items. It curtails energy production, increases inflammation, makes the body acidic, reduces immune function, raises blood pressure, alters brain chemistry, disrupts hormonal balance, and increases platelet stickiness. Stress even makes you fat—the stress hormone cortisol increases fat storage.

Many people stress themselves needlessly about things over which they have absolutely no control. Why do this? All it does is harm—to you! It's not worth the price. A woman once came to me for help for her cancer and numerous other health problems. I found out that twenty years prior she had gone through a nasty divorce. Then, every day for the past twenty years, she had relived the stress of that divorce—running the same movie over and over in her mind—the same high stress every day. Why? All it did was make her very sick.

Among other things, chronic stress interferes with normal hormonal signaling that controls inflammation, allowing inflammation to get out of control. Studies have shown that anger, fear, resentment, jealousy, and other "negative" emotions produce acidity in the body, while love, laughter, joy, and so on produce alkaline conditions.

Stress causes your body to release a flood of hormones into your blood. Hormones are part of your body's communications system, and they directly influence important cellular processes. For example, they deliver messages to genes and cells and act as genetic switches, turning genes on or off, including those that regulate cell growth, helping to protect against tumors.

Stress causes the release of growth-promoting hormones that help to switch cancer on and make it grow. Stress hormones also activate an inflammatory response, which promotes the growth and spread of tumors. Stress hormones make blood platelets sticky, causing them to form clots, contributing to strokes and heart attacks. At the same time, vital functions such as digestion, tissue repair, and immune response are put on hold and slowed down. In 1908 Dr. Eli Jones, in his book *Cancer: Its Causes, Symptoms, and Treatment*, said that stress is the number-one cause of cancer. Modern studies support his thinking. Patrick Quillin, Ph.D., in his book *Beating Cancer with Nutrition*, said, "In my years of experience, about 90% of the cancer patients I deal with have encountered a major traumatic event 1–2 years prior to the onset of cancer." The mind and the immune system are so intertwined that negative thinking depresses the activity of the immune system. When a person gives up and feels that life is no longer worth living, the immune system gives up as well.

In addition to switching cancer on, stress drives cancer. Norepinephrine, a hormone produced during periods of stress, increases the growth rate of cancer. Norepinephrine also stimulates tumor cells to release a chemical called *vascular endothelial growth factor*, which promotes growth of the blood vessels that feed growing tumors. The stress hormone epinephrine has been found to cause changes in prostate and breast cancer cells that make them resistant to the normal programmed cell death that prevents cancer.

Cortisol is another stress hormone. A study in a 2000 edition of the *Journal of the National Cancer Institute* measured survival in metastatic breast cancer patients and found that, up to seven years later, their daily cortisol levels were predictive of who would or would not survive. Cortisol and norepinephrine both block the action of cancer-protective natural killer cells. A study in the *Journal of Clinical Oncology* found that women with breast cancer who had positive attitudes had much more active natural killer cells than those who had sunk into depression and hopelessness.

Adrenaline is another hormone that we produce more of when we are stressed. Adrenaline depresses immunity by decreasing available antibodies and reducing the number and activity of lymphocytes. The membranes surrounding immune cells contain receptors for neurochemicals produced in the brain, so the brain is directly communicating with immune cells. When we are happy, the brain produces a type of neurochemical that causes the immune system to strengthen and build. When we are depressed, the brain produces another type of neurochemical that effectively shuts down the immune system.

This probably doesn't come as a surprise to those with pets, but research shows that cortisone and adrenaline are both reduced for pet owners. Owning a pet improves immune function, prevents heart attacks, cures depression, and helps you live longer. Numerous studies show that dogs can provide better stress relief and social support than friends and family; this lowers blood pressure, cholesterol, and triglycerides, and provides many other health benefits.

As the evidence builds, conventional medicine is finally beginning to understand how profoundly stress and negative thinking can harm your physical health, making you vulnerable to all kinds of health problems. There are good, scientifically sound reasons that people with positive outlooks live longer and healthier lives, while enjoying life far more than those with negative outlooks. Stress reduction techniques such as meditation are essential to preventing and healing disease.

The Choice Is Yours

One of the greatest gifts you can give yourself is to choose happiness. Too often we think that happiness is something that comes from outside us, but it really starts on the inside. Some people have every advantage in life and still are not happy. Wealth, status, and material goods do not create happiness. It is a positive attitude that matters. Older people with positive attitudes have a 55 percent lower risk of death from all causes. A study presented at the 2012 meeting of the American Society for Bone and Mineral Research showed that people with positive attitudes and purpose in life had the strongest bones. Your attitude is something you choose, and the more you stay genuinely positive, the better your health outcome is likely to be.

Many decades ago, I served a tour of duty in a U.S. Army combat infantry division. I knew from the nature of the job that I would be separated from friends and family, and that I would be facing stressful and unhappy experiences. The only real choice I had was to be unhappy or happy while experiencing them. I chose happy and happily lived through some very difficult situations. Your life is no different. You have to live it, and when life is filled with pain, sorrow, and disappointment, you can still choose to be happy regardless of the circumstances. Think about and be grateful for the blessings you do have; it's the choice that supports your immune system and your health. It's also more fun. Remember, happy comes from the inside, not the outside. It's a big mistake to depend on things outside of us for our happiness.

Once you make up your mind to be happy, life is better, and everything is easier. Admittedly, no one is going to be happy all the time, but if you choose to be happy, most of the time you will be. It will not only make you healthier but will help you get through even the worst of times. The more you smile, laugh, look on the bright side, and feel gratitude for what you have, the better your life will be. Wherever you go, bring your own sunshine.

One way to be happy is to have purpose in your life—following what motivates you and what makes you feel excited. Think about what gives you the most satisfaction and do something with it. Without purpose, life can be really dull, and your immune system will respond accordingly.

Knowing you can choose to be happy is liberating. You don't have to feel bad because you're getting older or your life isn't going exactly as you planned. Once you make your mind up to be happy, you actually don't have to feel bad for any reason.

Using Your Mind to Heal

The will to live is your most important medicine. A radical change in thought can create a radical change in your body. Remember, genes are obedient servants. The same gene can express in thousands of different ways, depending on what you ask it to do. When you change your thoughts, you change the instructions given to your genes, which changes how your genes express. The same genetic code you have always had will now be interpreted differently, which, for example, can mean the difference between having cancer or not having cancer.

In reality, when it comes to your potential for health, you are in the driver's seat. What it comes down to is two things—attention and intention. To affect the physical world, you have to pay attention to what it is you want to change and then give it the intention of how you would like it to change. This is the basis of the power of prayer. Spiritual practice has been known for millennia to bring about measurable changes in health. Dr. Larry Dossey, in his book *Healing Words*, describes the benefit of prayer as "one of the best-kept secrets in medical science." Dr. Dossey defines *prayerfulness* as a feeling of love, compassion, and empathy toward another, and he explains that prayer is a powerful and legitimate (if mostly overlooked) method of healing.

Numerous scientific experiments have now proven what many people have preached for thousands of years: attention and intention can change your physical world. Change is best achieved when people enter into a calm, meditative state and then focus their attention and intention on what they want. The meditative state is one in which normal thinking is suspended and you enter into the realm of pure awareness. If you haven't meditated in the past, it will take some practice to get rid of the mental chatter, quiet your mind and focus, and give attention to your intention. Learning how to meditate is a wise investment in your health and well-being.

Miracles can happen when people are in a calm mental and emotional state and apply attention and intention in order to change the physical world around them. In fact, tumors have been observed to shrink dramatically within hours when the patient is highly motivated. When you change your consciousness from one of disease to one of health, you can't lose.

During the depths of my illness, my body was progressively deteriorating. I realized that for survival, I needed to employ my mind as well as my body. I began quieting my mind and saying to myself over and over, "Every day, in every way, I get stronger and stronger and better and better." I kept repeating these words until I could feel strength coming into my body. I gave it a lot of attention and intention. At first, when I said this to myself, my mind fought back, saying, That's a lie! You feel worse today than you did yesterday. I realized my positive affirmations were being negated by my own thinking, so I began to reply to my mind by saying, "I know I feel worse today, but I am giving you an instruction."

Once I became comfortable giving my body instructions, my own objections began to disappear, and my body began to respond. I would say my affirmation, sometimes out loud, with passion and expectancy, many times daily. After a few weeks, my subconscious mind began to implement the instructions. One day, after saying these affirmations, I felt the best that I had felt since the onset of my illness more than a year before. The feeling lasted only five or ten minutes, but the fact that it happened proved I was on the right path. Soon the feelings of strength came more often and lasted longer. My badly damaged immune system was responding.

I began to understand that health and disease can be the reactions of the subconscious mind to the thoughts of the conscious mind; the subconscious takes orders from the conscious mind and implements them. Minds do what they are programmed to do, even though much of that programming is unintended. I began to realize my power to influence my health simply by choosing the daily thoughts I was putting into my mind. By focusing on my illness, I had been putting thoughts of disease into my mind, thereby creating more disease. The mind is always working, so why not make it work for rather than against you? Keep your images and suggestions as positive, simple, clear, and concise as possible.

Then repeat them as often as possible. Allow the subconscious to accept them as a command. When the mind speaks, the body listens.

Love, compassion, spiritual awareness, and all the life-affirming and positive emotions have extremely powerful implications for health. While these complex and nontangible concepts are often difficult to define, explain, or measure, they are perhaps the most real considerations in our lives. The will to live, choosing to be happy, and maintaining a state of inner peace and calm are keys to better health. In fact, there are recorded cures of cancer patients who did little more than change their diet and reduce their stress by meditating for a few hours every day. Ian Gawler, author of *You Can Conquer Cancer*, writes of his own personal experience with how his cancer was cured through meditation. Regular meditation is known to reduce stress, reduce inflammation, help regulate blood sugar levels, and enhance immune function. Each of these is vital to preventing or reversing any disease. Meditation is like a powerful magic elixir to improve your health, and it doesn't cost you anything.

Disease happens because the body is out of balance. The body has many natural rhythms, including something called heart rate variability. Regular meditation helps to normalize these biological rhythms, bringing the body back into balance and good health. When the body's rhythms are rebalanced, fewer inflammatory chemicals are produced, more anti-inflammatory chemicals are produced, and natural killer (NK) cell activity is enhanced. In truth, everyone should take time out to meditate every day. There are many good books on how to do this. What type of meditation you choose doesn't matter. Choose one that speaks to you, since they all take you to the same place and give you the same benefits.

Your mind is one of the most powerful tools of all, and it doesn't cost anything to use it. Put it to work and choose happy, loving thoughts and the belief that you will be well. Letting this seep into your subconscious through relaxed meditation can work miracles.

MAINTENANCE LIST
FOR MENTAL PATHWAY:

Energy Production

Avoid stress. It curtails energy production.

Inflammation

Avoid stress. It interferes with hormones that control inflammation.

Meditate regularly to rebalance the body's rhythms, which reduces inflammation.

Acid/Alkaline Balance

Avoid stress and negative emotions. They make your body acidic.

Digestive Health

Avoid generating stress hormones. They put digestion on hold or slow it down.

Hormonal Balance

Manage stress to minimize the release of cortisol, which disrupts hormonal balance.

Platelet Stickiness

Avoid releasing stress hormones. They make platelets sticky, causing blood clots.

Fat Storage

Stress hormones make you store fat.

Cultivate peace of mind, because stress and unhappiness can lead to overeating.

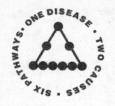

NINE

Physical Factors Affecting Your Health

Lack of activity destroys the good condition of every human being, while movement and methodical physical exercise save it and preserve it.

—Plato

Exposure to cell phone radiation is the largest human health experiment ever undertaken, without informed consent, and has some 4 billion participants enrolled. . . . I fear we will see a tsunami of brain tumors, although it is too early to see that now since the tumors have a thirty-year latency. I pray I'm wrong, but brace yourself.

—Lloyd Morgan, director, Central Brain
Tumor Registry of the United States, author of
Cell Phones and Brain Tumors: 15 Reasons for Concern

The Physical Pathway offers another opportunity to choose health. It involves the physical factors inside and outside your body, such as the health benefits you can reap by simply changing the way you breathe or by getting adequate sunlight. In this chapter I also give you alarming news about the harmful effects of everyday objects, like the dishwasher in your kitchen and the cell phone in your pocket. Use the Physical Pathway in the same way as the other pathways—as a guide to help you achieve a life free of disease.

What happens when we persistently use something in ways it's not designed to be used? Most of the time it will break down a lot faster than if we stick to the recommendations in the owner's manual. If we don't move, rest, and use our bodies the way they are meant to be used, we pay with damaged health. This chapter covers physical activities, like exercising, breathing, and sleeping, as well as elements of the physical environment—sunlight, electromagnetic fields, and noise—that impact your health.

Exercise

Exercise is one of the most effective medicines in the world—far more effective than prescription drugs. Many of today's health problems are linked to modern lifestyles that are simply incompatible with optimal biological functioning. We are the most sedentary people in history, yet it is a fact that an active lifestyle lowers the risk of getting sick and helps in getting well. As you now know, your health depends on giving your cells the nutrition they need and protecting them from toxins. However, here is another factor: *the need to move and stretch your cells.*

Moving and stretching cells facilitates the delivery of nutrients and the removal of toxins. Exercise is like a miracle drug; a 2013 study in the *British Medical Journal* concluded that exercise is more effective than frequently prescribed drugs. Movement is life. If you aren't moving, you are dying. In addition to helping deliver nutrients and promote detoxification, exercise balances hormones, reduces inflammation, and improves immune function. It fundamentally changes every system and function in your body. Exercise improves digestion, and a ten- to fifteen-minute walk after any meal has a beneficial effect on digestion. *Exercise is like an essential nutrient; if you don't get the amount you need, you will get sick.* Unfortunately, one in three Americans get little or no exercise at all.

While almost half of all Americans will develop cancer in their lifetime, only 14 percent of those who are physically active will develop cancer. Just thirty minutes of exercise every other day has been shown to cut the risk of breast cancer by 75 percent. A man's risk of prostate cancer is cut in half. Regular exercise has been shown to stimulate special cells in the brain, increasing their production of repair chemicals, protecting the brain from aging, and reducing the risk of cognitive decline. It actually triggers new brain cell growth in areas involved with higher mental function, making you smarter.

Exercise helps to provide oxygen to tissues. It helps to balance hormones by reducing the excess of estrogens and testosterone that are known to promote breast, prostate, uterine, ovarian, and testicular cancers. Exercise reduces insulin and blood sugar levels. Insulinlike growth factor (IGF), which contributes to inflammation and tumor growth, is also reduced. The amount of inflammatory cytokines in the blood is lowered with exercise, in turn lowering inflammation in the body. Exercise reduces platelet stickiness, reducing blood clot risk; it also increases the activity of clot-dissolving enzymes. By resetting the body's metabolism, exercise results in more fat burning. Exercise pumps the lymph system, improves lymph flow, and promotes the removal of toxic wastes from the body. In addition, exercise supports the immune system, stimulating natural killer (NK) cell activity, which is critical to preventing and curing cancer. *There isn't a drug or a medical treatment in the world that can do all this!* Best of all, this miracle treatment doesn't cost you a dime. The American Cancer Society recommends at least thirty minutes of moderate to vigorous physical activity five or more days a week.

While it's a good thing that you want to exercise, be careful where you exercise. Bicycling, jogging, or working out near a heavily traveled roadway can actually do more harm than your exercise is doing good. Studies show that exhaust fumes from cars and trucks cause health-damaging oxidative stress and inflammation throughout the body.

Historically, our daily survival required a lot of physical activity. Today we spend a lot of time sitting, and the latest research indicates that *even if you exercise regularly*, sitting for long stretches will make you sick. The lack of muscle contraction from lack of movement decreases blood flow throughout the body and reduces the efficiency of biological processes. In fact, sitting appears to be an independent risk factor for a variety of disease conditions. It's so bad that adults who spend an average of six hours a day watching television cut their life expectancy by five years. When doing prolonged sitting, regularly standing up is even more beneficial to health than continuing to sit and then doing regular walks.

All exercise is good, whether walking, swimming, or tennis, but with our busy lifestyles, many people say they can't find the time to exercise. Fortunately, there is a way to cheat—an extremely effective form of exercise that anyone can do at home. *Rebounding* is a type of exercise that involves bouncing up and down on a mini-trampoline, and its effects are almost magical. Simple, surprisingly easy to do, safe, and a lot of fun, rebounding can be done by almost anyone, regardless of age or physical condition. You can rebound while you watch TV or even while talking on the telephone. Get up from your desk or the couch every half hour and rebound for a couple of minutes. Rebounding tones, conditions, strengthens, and heals the entire body in as little as fifteen minutes per day—more is better.

Jumping up and down on a rebounder moves and stretches every cell in your body simultaneously, so it is a concentrated form of exercise. When you bounce on a rebounder, your entire body (internal organs, bones, connective tissue, and skin) becomes stronger, more flexible, and healthier. Blood circulation, oxygen delivery, lymphatic drainage, and toxin removal are vastly improved.

Rebounding alternately puts pressure on and takes pressure off body cells, like squeezing a sponge. This moving and stretching of the cells facilitates nutrient delivery and toxin removal, which is exactly what you need to be healthy. Rebounding gives you all of this without having to take the time to go to the gym, work up a sweat, or end up with sore muscles and possible injuries. One caveat is that poor-quality rebounders may shock the joints and tissues and cause injury. Look for barrel springs that are fatter in the middle and tapered at the ends. (See Appendix A for assistance.)

The good news is that studies show that a modest amount of exercise, even fifteen minutes a day, can increase your life span and reduce all-cause mortality. On the other hand, every hour spent sitting reduces life expectancy, comparable with other major risk factors, such as obesity. Exercise is an amazing wonder drug!

Breathing

Oxygen is our most critical nutrient. We can live only minutes without it. Getting the oxygen we need depends on numerous factors, including how we breathe. Failure to breathe correctly deprives our cells of needed oxygen and changes body chemistry. Deep breathing supplies more oxygen, and shallow breathing less. Most of us do shallow breathing.

Just as we can control what foods we eat, the toxins we are exposed to, the thoughts we put into our mind, and how much exercise we get, we can also control how we breathe and how much oxygen we supply to our bodies. The way you breathe can substantially affect how you look and feel, your resistance to disease, and even how long you live. Proper breathing technique helps to optimize your health as well as keep you relaxed and more mentally alert.

We are all born knowing how to breathe correctly, but the stress of modern living has caused many people to develop poor breathing habits. The most common problem is shallow or rapid breathing, also called overbreathing. Despite the name, overbreathing actually results in less oxygen being available to cells. Overbreathing is usually caused by stress, and it manifests as shallow chest breathing, irregular breathing, rapid breathing, or holding of the breath. On occasion, overbreathing is not a problem, and we all do it, but many of us breathe too rapidly all the time. We breathe more times per minute than we should and take breaths that are too shallow.

Overbreathing not only causes an oxygen deficiency, it also causes a carbon dioxide deficiency. Rapid breathing causes the body to lose too much carbon dioxide; the body needs to maintain normal levels of both oxygen and carbon dioxide. Oxygen is transported to tissues by bonding with hemoglobin in red blood cells. Normal oxygen respiration creates carbon dioxide as a metabolic waste product. Local concentrations of carbon dioxide signal the red blood cells to release their oxygen so that your cells can obtain a new supply of oxygen. When you expel too much carbon dioxide through rapid breathing, insufficient carbon dioxide is present to cause the hemoglobin to release its oxygen. Your cells and tissues then become oxygen-deficient. In addition, insufficient carbon dioxide changes the pH of the blood, causing a loss of alkaline minerals and contributing to osteoporosis.

To breathe correctly, bring air down into the lungs by using the diaphragm, a deep abdominal muscle that nature intended for breathing. Breathing downward with the diaphragm (belly breathing instead of chest breathing) is an effortless and efficient way to breathe. Unfortunately, people often use their chest and upper back to breathe; chest breathing takes more effort and is less efficient. Breathing downward with the diaphragm (as opposed to outward with the chest) moves the viscera (guts) down and away, making more room for the lungs and creating the capacity for more air in your lungs and more oxygen for your tissues, whether you are exercising or at rest. Each breath should begin downward in the belly, only moving up into the chest when necessary. Correct breathing should be effortless, through the nose rather than mouth, and relatively slow—at a resting rate of less than fifteen breaths per minute, preferably eight to ten. The way we breathe has such profound effects, both physically and psychologically, it is little surprise that many ancient traditions—such as meditation, yoga, and martial arts— rely first and foremost on breathing technique. Daily deep breathing exercises are very calming and help to keep you oxygenated and healthy.

Sunlight

Sunlight is like an essential nutrient and a magic elixir for the body. It's one of nature's most powerful healing agents and goes way beyond the benefits of creating vitamin D. Our ancestors were out in the sun all the time, and cancer was a rare disease. Yet we are advised to avoid the sun, and cancer is epidemic. This bad advice has created an epidemic of vitamin D deficiency, costing countless thousands of lives from vitamin D–deficiency diseases such as heart disease, multiple sclerosis, osteoporosis, type 1 diabetes, infections, autoimmune diseases, depression, asthma, and cancer. Science doesn't even begin to understand all the marvelous benefits of sunlight, yet the disease industry continues to perpetuate the myth that the sun causes cancer. Exactly the opposite is true. Cells have light-activated receptors that, when triggered, initiate a number of beneficial and cancer-protective biological reactions. Sunlight has a beneficial effect on platelet stickiness and helps to prevent blood clots. Sunlight also affects cell membrane electrons, helping to charge your batteries and energize your body.

Vitamin D plays a critical role in preventing cancer. It is one of our most important nutrients, and about 90 percent of our vitamin D comes from the interaction of sunlight with cholesterol-like compounds in our skin. If sunlight were bad for us, why would Mother Nature make us dependent on it? We are designed to need sunlight, and the more sunlight you get, the healthier you will be. In fact, because people who live in the northern latitudes get less sunlight, they get more cancer. Northerners get more of all kinds of vitamin D–deficiency diseases. More than 40 percent of the U.S. population is vitamin D deficient, and that can go up to 75 percent by the end of the winter. Vitamin D is crucial to immune function, and flu spreads quickly in the winter because people are vitamin D deficient.

Vitamin D acts like a hormone and interacts with genes, giving them crucial instructions that prevent cancer. Without sufficient vitamin D, the risk of cancer skyrockets. Research indicates that people with the lowest blood levels of vitamin D are four times more likely to die of colon cancer. A 2008 study in *Carcinogenesis* found that women with breast cancer were three times more likely to have low vitamin D levels.

Caution: The fact that sunlight is necessary for health is not an invitation to rush out and get sunburned. Sunburn damages DNA and can cause cancer. Too much of a good thing can be bad for you. People with light skin need less sunlight than those with dark skin. In fact, people with dark skin need a lot more sunlight to get the same benefits. Use the sun sensibly. Don't abuse it, and it will be your partner in health. Best is to get sun as often as possible in small, graduated doses. When outdoors for long periods, wear protective clothing and a wide-brimmed hat.

Research shows that sunlight nourishes and energizes the human body, helping in the prevention of infections from bacteria, molds, and viruses. Sunlight helps to regulate hormones and stimulates the production of melatonin and testosterone. Sunlight enhances the immune system by increasing white blood cell count as well as gamma globulin, a protein that helps the body fight infection. Significantly, sunlight stimulates the production of more red blood cells, increasing the oxygen content of the blood, which helps to prevent and reverse cancer.

Sunlight is also good for the heart. It enables the body to lower the resting pulse rate, lower blood pressure, and lower cholesterol as well as triglycerides in the blood. In fact, sunlight may decrease cholesterol by more than 30 percent. It also enhances the power of the skin to resist diseases such as psoriasis, eczema, and acne. Sunlight lowers blood sugar and enhances liver function as well. It stimulates the liver to produce an enzyme that increases your ability to detoxify environmental pollutants. Further, sunlight stimulates the pineal gland to produce vital brain chemicals such as tryptamines, which cheer you up and prevent anxiety and depression.

Do not use sunscreens! Sunscreens are neither beneficial nor safe. They block out essential wavelengths that the body needs. Most sunscreen products contain numerous toxic chemicals, some of which can even cause cancer. Further, sunscreens contain aluminum nanoparticles. These nanoparticles get into the body and damage mitochondria, severely depleting ATP production and reducing your energy supply. Dating from antiquity, approaches to protecting against sun damage have included using high-quality olive oil or coconut oil on the skin.

Electromagnetic Fields

The human body is a battery-operated electronic device. Each of our trillions of cells produce their own magnetic fields and communicate via electromagnetic frequencies. Cell membranes act as semiconductors, diodes, microprocessors, and capacitors to store voltage. Every organ in the body produces its own unique electromagnetic field.

Disturbing your electromagnetic balance affects your health, and a growing body of evidence indicates that brain cancer is only one of the many health problems that our new wireless society is producing. Invisible to the human eye, electromagnetic fields (EMFs) are present everywhere in our environment. The body's electromagnetic field and its electrical system are affected by the external EMFs, increasingly coming from Wi-Fi networks, cordless phones, cell phones, and cell phone towers. Over the last century, exposure to man-made EMFs has been increasing steadily as growing demand for electricity, ever-advancing technologies, and changes in social behavior have created more and more artificial sources. At home and at work, from the generation and transmission of electricity, to domestic appliances and industrial equipment, to telecommunications and broadcasting, all of us are now exposed to a complex mix of electric and magnetic fields.

Increasingly, people are becoming electromagnetically sensitive. An estimated 5 percent of the population in developed countries now experience serious electrohypersensitivity symptoms, while 35 percent experience mild symptoms. Some people can be totally debilitated just by walking into a Wi-Fi–equipped area. One symptom of electrohypersensitivity is altered sugar metabolism similar to diabetes. In fact, some researchers believe we have a new kind of diabetes caused by electromagnetic sensitivity. A study in a 2010 issue of *Electromagnetic Health* found that cordless phones can interfere with your heart, causing abnormal rhythms. Dr.

Thomas Rau, medical director of the world-renowned Paracelsus Clinic in Switzerland, says he is convinced that electromagnetic loads lead to concentration problems, ADD, tinnitus, migraines, insomnia, arrhythmia, Parkinson's, and cancer.

Given that the body is a battery-operated electronic device, no one who understands this will question whether external electromagnetic fields are affecting us. The only real question is how much harm they are doing.

Power Lines

A 2007 study in the *Internal Medicine Journal* found that living next to high-voltage power lines increased the risk of cancer. People who lived within 328 yards of a power line up to age five were five times more likely to develop cancer. In addition, children who lived that close to a power line at any point during their first fifteen years were three times more likely to develop cancer as adults. The study concluded that living for a prolonged period near high-voltage power lines is likely to increase the risk of leukemia, lymphoma, and other cancers later in life. The power industry had previously dismissed safety concerns after studies failed to show increased cases of leukemia in children living near power lines. This 2007 study is significant and alarming because it shows that, while the children didn't get cancer, their exposure had long-lasting effects and the cancer shows up in adults who were exposed as children. Based on this study and others, it would be prudent not to live, work, or go to school within 300 yards of a high-voltage power line.

Cell Phones

EMFs present challenges for those wishing to stay healthy. We are all exposed to EMFs in our daily living. We can't escape them because electromagnetic pollution is the single largest change we have made to our environment. Cell phones, computer screens, TV sets, hair dryers, refrigerators, dishwashers, and even the clock radio by the side of your bed are putting out unhealthy levels of EMFs. Driving your car exposes you to a lot of EMFs. While we have little personal control over many of the EMFs in our environment, such as radio and TV broadcasts, we have a lot of control over some of them. Cell phone use is one example. *A Swedish study has found that heavy users of cell phones had a 240 percent increase in brain tumors on the sides of their heads on which the phones were used.* This is a good reason to limit cell phone use and to use the speakerphone option to avoid holding the phone next to your head. In 2007 the European Union's environmental watchdog agency warned that cell phone technology "could lead to a health crisis similar to those caused by asbestos, smoking, and lead in petrol."

Tragically, children and teens are using cell phones. In the United States, 90 percent of sixteen-year-olds have their own cell phones, as do many primary school children. It is noteworthy that brain cancer has now surpassed leukemia as the number-one cancer killer in children. The incidence of pediatric brain cancers in Australia increased 21 percent in just one decade.

Because the negative effects of cell phone usage are not immediate, people think cell phones are safe. While cell phones have been used heavily for about twenty years, it can take up to thirty years for brain tumors to develop as a result of their use. Children, however, are more susceptible to cell phone damage because their cells are still reproducing more rapidly. Their brains and nervous systems are still developing, and their skulls are thinner. A study by Dr. Lennart Hardell, a professor of oncology and cancer epidemiology in Sweden, found that teenagers who use cell phones heavily have 500 percent more brain cancer as young adults. The study also found that the risk for young people who used cordless phones was almost as great, at more than 400 percent higher than those who avoided their use. In Europe and the United Kingdom, the incidence of brain tumors has increased by 40 percent over the last twenty years. Some researchers are predicting an epidemic of brain cancer as cell phone use continues to grow. Here is what Dr. Hardell had to say about cell phone use in a July 2003 interview on *60 Minutes:*

> *What we did find was an increased risk for tumors in the temporal area of the brain, which is that part of the brain where the highest exposure to microwaves on the same side as the person had used the mobile phone. We found overall an increased risk of 30 percent for brain tumors, increasing for those who had used the mobile phone for over 10 years to 80 percent increased risk. This is a significant finding.*

One of the largest studies ever, the Interphone study, involving thirteen countries, found a 300 percent increased risk of acoustic nerve tumors, and an increased risk of tumors of the parotid salivary gland, owing to cell phone use. An Israeli scientist, Dr. Siegal Sadetzki, concluded in an *American Journal of Epidemiology* study that there is a link between cell phone usage and the development of cancer of the salivary glands. Other studies have indicated risks beyond brain and salivary tumors, finding cognitive problems, disorientation, eye damage, bone damage, Alzheimer's, and others. A 2002 study in *Epidemiology* and a 1998 study in *Lancet* found that cell phone radiation causes miscarriages and increases blood pressure.

Research sponsored by the telecommunications industry found an almost 300 percent increase in the incidence of genetic damage when human blood cells were exposed to cell phone radiation. Dr. Ronald B. Herberman, the head of the University of Pittsburgh Cancer Institute, advises against using cell phones in public places because it exposes other people to the hazardous EMFs that you are generating. Cell phones not only affect the user but, like secondhand smoke, also affect those around the user. Even being more than ten feet away from a cell phone user modifies your brain wave patterns, affects your short-term memory, and even affects your ability to perform physical tasks such as driving a car. In 2009 Dr. Herberman issued an unprecedented warning to his faculty and staff: Limit cell phone use because of the health risks. Students with the highest frequency of cell phone use have lower grade point averages, experience more anxiety, and are less happy than peers who used cell phones less often.

Children especially should be protected from this EMF pollution; cell phones should not be used in close proximity to children. Lloyd Morgan, a director of the Central Brain Tumor Registry of the United States, had this to say: "Exposure to cell phone radiation is the largest human health experiment ever undertaken, without informed consent, and has some 4 billion participants enrolled. I fear we will see a tsunami of brain tumors, although it is too early to see that now since the tumors have a thirty-year latency. I pray I'm wrong, but brace yourself."

Studies in other nations confirm that living close to cell phone towers damages health. People living close to these transmitters suffered extreme sleep disruption, chronic fatigue, nausea, skin problems, irritability, brain disturbances, and cardiovascular problems. German researchers found that people living within 1,200 feet of a cell tower experienced high cancer rates and developed their tumors on average eight years earlier than the national average. Breast cancer topped the list. Spanish researchers found that people living within 1,000 feet of cellular antennas developed illnesses at average power densities thousands of times lower than those allowed by international exposure standards. Researchers in Israel found that people who lived near a cell tower for three to seven years had a cancer rate four times higher than the control population.

Rooftop transmitters, which readily pass microwave radiation into structures, can be especially dangerous. Across the world there are reports of cancer clusters and extreme illness in office buildings and multitenant dwellings where antennas are placed on rooftops directly over workers and tenants. In 2006 the top floors of a Melbourne University office building were closed after a brain tumor cluster drew media attention to the risks of cell phone towers on top of the building.

Wi-Fi

Countless Wi-Fi systems, indoors and out, accommodate wireless laptop computers, personal digital assistants, Wi-Fi–enabled phones, gaming devices, video cameras, even parking and utility meters. Hundreds of cities already have or are planning to fund Wi-Fi networks, each consisting of thousands of small microwave transmitters bolted to buildings, street lamps, park benches, and bus stops, and even buried under sidewalks. All this has been planned with virtually no studies or warning signs about radiation exposure. Not a single environmental or public health study has been required as the industry unleashes this new wireless technology from which no living thing will escape.

Dr. Robert Becker, noted for decades of research on the effects of electromagnetic radiation, has warned, "Even if we survive the chemical and atomic threats to our existence, there is the strong possibility that increasing electropollution could set in motion irreversible changes leading to our extinction before we are even aware of them."

Good Advice

To protect your health, limit your cell phone use to only the most essential calls, and then limit the call to less than two minutes. Cell phones are a fact of life. They aren't going to go away. The challenge is to use them as safely as possible. Make no nonessential phone calls. When cell phones are on, they are emitting radiation, even when you are not using them. Do not carry a cell phone close to your body while it is on. Keep your phone turned off when it is not being used; turn it on as needed to check for messages. Do not hold a phone next to your brain. Use the speakerphone feature to make your calls, keeping the phone as far away as possible. Keep children away from the immediate vicinity when you make a call. Do not allow children under the age of eighteen to use a cell phone except in emergencies. Use of cell phones inside buildings, aircraft, or in cars increases cancer risk, because it increases the radiation a phone must emit in order to function. Don't live within 1,200 feet of a cell phone antenna. Use of text messages and nonwireless headsets can reduce, but not eliminate, cancer risk. The evidence is becoming overwhelming that cell phone use is hazardous to your health, but do not count on the government to protect you. Federal exposure limits have been deliberately set so high that no matter how much additional wireless radiation is added to the national burden, it will always be "within standards."

When buying a home or choosing an apartment, choose one that is not immediately adjacent to high-voltage transmission lines, cell phone towers, or transformers. Be prudent in the use of appliances. When possible, use rechargeable battery-powered appliances rather than plug-in models. Do not stand immediately next to an electrical appliance when it is turned on. Turn on the dishwasher when finished in the kitchen and you are ready to leave the room. Avoid electric blankets or use them only to warm up the bed before you get in it. Keep telephone answering machines and electric clocks away from your head while you are sleeping. Increase distance from televisions (at least six feet away) and avoid appliances that come into close contact with your body such as hairdryers and nonbattery electric razors.

Airport Scanners

Another hazard worthy of special note is the body scanners used to screen passengers in airports. One type of scanner uses x-rays, and it is a well-established fact that the ionizing radiation of x-rays damages DNA and causes cancer. However, another type of scanner uses a technology called *terahertz waves* (THz waves). THz waves are thought to be safe because they do not have the energy of x-rays and are not ionizing. However, while the energy of THz waves is low and nonionizing, research at the Center for Nonlinear Studies at Los Alamos National Laboratory in New Mexico raises questions. These waves may interact with double-stranded DNA in a novel way. They produce resonant forces that unzip the strands of the DNA, doing catastrophic damage, interfering with gene expression and DNA replication. No one knows what the effects may be. Given these facts, being bombarded by THz waves in every airport is probably not a good idea.

While these scanners may be good for security, they are not good for your health. To be safe, refuse to go through airport scanners. This will subject you to the inconvenience of a personal search, but the inconvenience is better than the unknown consequences of the damage the scanners can cause.

Sleep

Getting a good night's sleep is essential to good health and another piece of the puzzle to preventing disease or restoring health. The body is designed for certain sleep patterns, and disturbing those patterns can seriously alter the balance of hormones in your body. The reality is that our bodies have been programmed over millennia to sleep when it's dark and be awake during daylight. This is how our ancestors lived, and when you do otherwise, you are sending conflicting signals to the body. This upsets normal biochemistry and balance, creating disease. We know that sleep affects immunity, blood pressure, diabetes, and even obesity.

Unfortunately, a good night's sleep is increasingly losing out to late-night TV, the Internet, emails, and the other distractions of modern life. According to a poll by the National Sleep Foundation, the majority of Americans are not getting enough sleep. Only 40 percent of the respondents reported getting a good night's sleep every night or almost every night. Lawrence Epstein, president of the American Academy of Sleep Medicine, said, "We have in our society this idea that you can just get by without sleep or manipulate when you sleep without any consequences. What we're finding is that's just not true."

The amount of necessary sleep varies from person to person. Most people need between seven and nine hours. Research indicates that sleeping less than eight hours a night has significant cumulative consequences.

People who get less than six hours are at greatly increased risk for disease. A study by Harvard Medical School of over 82,000 nurses found that getting less than six hours sleep per night increases the risk of premature death. Links have also been discovered between too little sleep and diabetes, obesity, hypertension, and high cholesterol. Surprisingly, there was also a risk of premature death for those sleeping more than nine hours.

The picture that is emerging is that not sleeping enough, being awake in the early-morning hours, or waking up frequently at night throws the body's internal clock out of whack. "Lack of sleep disrupts every physiologic function in the body," said Dr. Eve Van Cauter of the University of Chicago. "We have nothing in our biology that allows us to adapt to this behavior."

Sleep regulates hormonal balance, and hormonal balance is essential to health. Studies indicate that lack of sleep increases the production of stress hormones, and stress hormones both cause and drive cancer. Cortisol is one of the hormones affected. Cortisol helps to regulate the release of natural killer cells that help the body battle cancer. Cortisol needs to be properly balanced, but night shift workers have a shifted cortisol balance. People who wake up frequently during the night are also more likely to have abnormal cortisol rhythms that throw the body out of balance.

Melatonin is another hormone affected by sleep. This hormone is produced in the brain during sleep; it helps people fall asleep faster and stay asleep, experience less restlessness, and prevent daytime fatigue. It boosts the immune system. Melatonin provides powerful anticancer benefits and interferes with tumor growth. Melatonin is a powerful antioxidant, helping protect DNA from cancer-causing mutations. However, melatonin production is sensitive to the amount of sleep we get and the amount of light we are exposed to. This has become a problem, especially with the exploding number of artificial light-producing electrical gadgets that are now part of our daily lives. Many people keep these devices in close proximity during night hours and are continually exposed to light emissions during sleep that reduce melatonin production. A wealth of research is indicating an increasing risk of cancer as a result.

Research shows that even the smallest amount of light from devices such as iPods, laptops, electronic readers, and TV sets is sufficient to cut melatonin production in half. This emphasizes the importance of sleeping in a totally dark room to lower cancer risk. Electromagnetic fields (EMFs) in the bedroom can also disrupt melatonin production. You can purchase a gauss meter to measure EMF levels in various parts of your home. Move all electrical devices at least three feet from your bed. Shift workers who are up all night produce less melatonin. This is why the World Health Organization has labeled this kind of work a "probable carcinogen."

Insufficient melatonin affects levels of other hormones and increases estrogen. High estrogen increases the risk of breast and prostate cancer. The truth is that even minimal exposure to an artificial light source is sufficient to alter the expression of genes that are connected to the formation of cancer as well as of genes that assist in the fight against cancer. When melatonin production is delayed or halted by artificial light sources, our nighttime rhythms are disturbed, and normal metabolic activity required for cellular repair is disrupted. The body requires seven to nine hours of uninterrupted sleep each night, with no light distraction, to complete the repair functions that are essential to maintaining optimal health.

Interfering with the body's natural rhythms is never a good idea. Health is when the body is balanced and functioning normally. Female night-shift workers have higher rates of breast cancer than women who sleep normal hours, and they are more likely to have more rapid tumor growth and to die earlier from breast cancer. Tumors grow two to three times faster in laboratory animals with severe sleep dysfunctions. Sleep helps to restore one's internal environment, and people who sleep poorly or do not get enough sleep have higher levels of inflammation. Getting six or fewer hours of sleep increases levels of three inflammatory markers: fibrinogen, IL-6, and C-reactive protein, resulting in chronic low-grade inflammation.

Cell phones are another problem affecting sleep. A Swedish study published by MIT's Progress in Electromagnetics Research Symposium said there was now "more than sufficient evidence" to show that cell phone radiation delays and reduces sleep. Using cell phones before bed causes people to take longer to reach the deeper stages of sleep and to spend less time in them. Less time in the deeper stages of sleep interferes with the body's ability to do its daily repairs. Repair deficits impair your immune system, leaving you less able to fight off diseases of all kinds, as well as contributing to the aging process. Adequate sleep is one of the most important factors in your health and quality of life.

Noise

Noise can kill! Research has proven that noise can cause serious health problems. Chronic noise raises the level of stress hormones and substantially increases the risk of heart attack, high blood pressure, and stroke. Exposure to high levels of aircraft noise increases risk of cardiovascular disease. Noise has been linked to cancer through disrupted sleep patterns and the resulting hormonal imbalances. Everything from aircraft traffic to barking dogs and loud music can interrupt sleep patterns and result in abnormal hormone secretions. Disrupted hormonal balance creates abnormal immune responses, resulting in cancer-supporting conditions. The problems caused by noise go beyond sleep loss. Workers chronically exposed to loud noise suffered calcium and magnesium losses, which can affect a variety of health problems, from osteoporosis to cancer.

The body reacts to noise by secreting inflammatory chemicals (cytokines). Some researchers believe that one reason cytokine production rises as we grow older is exposure to a lifetime of noise. The bottom line is that noise disrupts normal hormonal balance and normal immune response, and creates inflammation in the body. Inflammation is the foundation of every chronic disease. As much as possible, reduce the amount of noise in your life.

Things to Remember

Many factors affect our overall health, and the factors in the Physical Pathway are among them. By controlling these factors in your favor, as well as those in the other five of the Six Pathways, you can move yourself toward a disease-free life.

- Be sure to get at least thirty minutes of exercise every other day at a minimum.
- Rebounding even twenty minutes a day as you watch TV or listen to music will do wonders for your health, and at no inconvenience.
- Watch your breathing throughout the day. Proper breathing will help you relax, lower your stress levels, and supply more oxygen to your cells.
- Get frequent sunlight on most of your body. When this is not possible, be sure to take a high-quality vitamin D supplement.
- Minimize your exposure to radiation of all kinds, from medical x-rays to cell phones to airport scanners.
- Go to bed before 11 PM and try to get eight hours of sleep every night.
- Avoid noise, especially chronic, loud noise.

YOUR MAINTENANCE LIST FOR THE PHYSICAL PATHWAY:

Energy Production

Exercise helps oxygenate cells and tissues, increasing energy production.

Sunlight helps to charge your batteries and energize your body.

Inflammation

Get enough sleep. Lack of sleep increases inflammation.

Chronic noise causes the body to secrete inflammatory chemicals.

Get your body moving. Exercise reduces inflammation in many different ways.

Avoid vehicle exhaust fumes. They cause oxidative stress and inflammation.

Acid/Alkaline Balance

Breathe slowly and deeply. Overbreathing can upset your pH balance.

Digestive Health

Walking ten to fifteen minutes after any meal improves digestion.

Hormonal Balance

Get a good night's sleep every night. Sleep regulates hormonal balance.

Avoid chronic exposure to noise. It raises the level of stress hormones.

Get regular exercise. It helps to balance hormones.

Sunlight helps to regulate hormones and stimulates the production of melatonin and testosterone.

Platelet Stickiness

Exercise reduces platelet stickiness, reducing blood clot risk.

Exercise increases the activity of clot-dissolving enzymes.

Sunlight has a beneficial effect on platelet stickiness, helping to prevent clots.

Fat Storage

Exercise resets the body's metabolism, causing it to burn more fat.

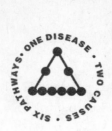

TEN

It's Not in Your Genes

Nutrition can alter the course of high-risk genes,
not only by turning these genes off but also by inhibiting
the resulting bad effects produced by them.

—Russell L. Blaylock, M.D.,
Health and Nutrition Secrets

Genetics may load the gun,
but environment pulls the trigger.

—Pamela Peeke, M.D., M.P.H.

Understanding Genes

There is an enormous amount of misunderstanding about genes. This Genetic Pathway chapter will help clear up this misunderstanding and open up new possibilities for you. Our physicians blame everything on age, germs, and genes. Wrong on all counts! It is possible to live to a very old age in perfect health, so age alone does not cause disease. We live in a sea of germs. If germs caused disease, we would all be dead. It is we who cause infections by compromising our immunity and upsetting the balance between ourselves and the microbes in our environment. It's the same problem with genes. With very few exceptions, genes don't cause disease. All of us have genetic predispositions to certain ailments, but that doesn't mean we will develop those problems. In order to get the ailment, specific genes have to be activated and express in a certain way. So don't activate them! You are in charge. *Genes run our lives, but we run the genes, so we run our lives.*

Within each of our trillions of microscopic cells is a nucleus that contains a set of instructions we call *genes*. Every cell in your body contains about 30,000 genes, and these determine the color of your eyes, the color of your hair, whether you have long or short legs, and many other physical traits. We inherit these genetic instructions from our parents, and they govern how we look and how our body works.

But only about one-quarter of our genes express (turn on) automatically, determining, for example, whether our eyes are blue or our hair is curly. Most genes merely offer thousands of possibilities—what *can* happen, not what *will* happen. If certain circumstances are present, then certain genes will express in a particular way—perhaps a healthy way. If other circumstances are present, those same genes will express in a different way—perhaps an unhealthy way. By themselves, genes do not determine our sickness or health. *It's the instructions the genes receive that are most responsible for our health and performance.* We are not taught this fact.

Some people have an abnormal BRCA gene (which increases the risk of breast cancer), but it does not mean they will get breast cancer. Most people with this abnormality do *not* get cancer. It is merely a possibility—unless they cause the gene to express in a way that makes it a reality.

Similar to a program on your computer, genes offer a range of options of what you can do within that program. But they need an instruction, some sort of a trigger—environmental or psychological—for them to choose which option to express. You are in control of these triggers through your diet, lifestyle, and thoughts. *There isn't a single pharmaceutical that can up-regulate gene expression.* Yet gene expression in well over 500 genes can be enhanced, to maintain and create health, with simple changes in diet and lifestyle.

Different cellular environments give different instructions to genes. By changing the environment—for example, your pH—you change how the genes function and consequently how you function. The chemical environment you create in your cells by what you eat, the toxins you are exposed to, and your thoughts provides instructions for the genes.

Genes are also living structures, susceptible to damage, mutation, and repair, as well as to the instructions you give to them.

You Control Your Genes

We worry far more than we need to about genetic inheritance. Following the advent of human genome sequencing, scientists have redoubled their efforts to isolate "disease genes." Numerous papers have been published holding out distant hope for "genetic therapies" for everything from wrinkles to heart disease. However, what you really need to know about health is that you can stay well or get well with the genes you have. Are there genes that make you more susceptible to Alzheimer's and heart conditions? No doubt. Will these genes cause these diseases? No! To cause disease, you have to turn off protective genes, activate disease-promoting genes, and then drive the disease process. Consider that a century ago cancer affected only 3 percent of the American population. Now almost half of all Americans will develop cancer in their lifetimes. Our genes haven't changed in the last century, but our diet, environment, and lifestyle have. We cannot blame our epidemic of degenerative diseases and premature aging on inherited genes. *The real problem is that we are giving them the wrong instructions and doing unprecedented damage to our genes as well.*

Genes are obedient servants, and they do what we ask them to do. Unfortunately, in today's world, we are asking our genes to make us sick. We are damaging our genes, giving them improper instructions, and in every way possible causing them to malfunction. Through our nutritionally deficient diet, exposure to toxins, exposure to radiation, stress, lack of sleep, and other factors, not only are we instructing our genes to make us sick, but we are also shutting down the DNA repair genes that are there to protect us from premature aging and disease. We are doing everything just right to get old and sick.

To get well and stay well, you have to:

• Stop damaging your genes.
• Support DNA repair.
• Give your genes the correct instructions.

To get well and stay well, the most promising genetic therapy is to spare your genes the constant onslaught of nutritional deficiencies, toxins, stress, and radiation. The environment we create for our genes is a trigger that causes genes to express in different ways, and you are creating that environment every moment of every day with the foods you eat, the air you breathe, the water you drink, and the thoughts you think. When you do this right, you will maintain normal chemistry in your cells. Normal chemistry gives genes healthy instructions, keeping disease turned off.

Give Correct Instructions to Your Genes

When turned on, a single gene is capable of producing many thousands of different proteins. Each protein creates a different outcome, and if you want a health-supporting outcome, you have to produce the correct protein. Which protein out of the thousands of possibilities the gene will actually produce depends on the instructions it receives from its environment—which you create. For example, a study of twins reported in a 2000 *New England Journal of Medicine* concluded, "The overwhelming contributor to the causation of cancer in the populations of twins that we studied was the environment." A 2011 doctoral dissertation by John D. Clarke, a molecular and cellular biologist, proved that a diet rich in broccoli sprouts was able to prevent prostate cancer. Dr. Terry Wahls, M.D., was able to reverse her multiple sclerosis without pharmaceuticals by eating a diet high in organic sulfur-rich foods, including broccoli. Eating nutritious foods created a different chemical environment in the cells, giving different instructions to the genes, both preventing and curing disease.

The chemical environment you create inside each cell depends on your nutrition, your level of physical activity; the amount of sunlight, fresh air, and sleep you get; the pH and amount of sodium inside your cells; the amount and kind of toxins in your cells; the hormones and hormonelike chemicals you have consumed; the electromagnetic environment you're exposed to; and your thoughts, beliefs, and emotions. One way or another, all this is under your control.

Hormones are genetic switches, activating certain genes and deactivating others. It is extremely important to your health that you normalize hormone function. Hormonal balance is why getting the right amount of sleep is so important and why stress hormones can kill you.

One reason that sugar is such a dangerous toxin is that it unbalances your hormones. It is also why consuming hormones contained in meat and dairy products causes disease.

Nutrients in your diet interact with your genes. Scientists have discovered that vitamin D directly influences over 200 genes. Included are genes connected to cancer and autoimmune diseases like multiple sclerosis. Availability of vitamin D at a critical time can mean the difference between a debilitating illness and excellent health. By the end of winter, most Americans are vitamin D deficient.

Sleep affects how your genes will express. A 2013 study in the *Proceedings of the National Academy of Sciences* found that sleeping less than six hours a night affects the activity of over 700 genes. Even one week of insufficient sleep will cause abnormal gene expression in blood cells and disrupt normal body rhythms. The genes that were affected are responsible for controlling immunity, inflammation, and our response to stress.

Studies of cancer patients have shown that lifestyle changes involving diet, exercise, and human interaction can alter the expression of hundreds of cancer-related genes in the direction of health. Meanwhile, stress hormones have been found to change gene expression for the worse. Stress hormones affect virtually every cell in the body, and the negative programming can remain even after the hormones have returned to their normal levels. Whether you are mentally stressed or able to maintain a more positive outlook can influence the expression of your genes and thus directly impact your health and biological age.

Regular exercise has been found to alter the expression of over 7,000 genes—an enormous impact. Genes that control obesity, type 2 diabetes, and fat storage are all changed for the better by exercising regularly.

Gene Mutations
Damage Your Health

Mutations caused by malnutrition, toxins, and radiation can cause dramatic and unpredictable changes in genetic coding. Making random coding changes to a computer program creates chaos, and the same thing happens when you create random coding changes in your genes.

You must do everything you can to protect yourself from DNA mutations, which means eating a good diet and limiting your exposure to DNA-damaging toxins and radiation. As we age, our DNA repair capability is reduced, and it becomes all the more important to protect your DNA from damage. Here are some considerations:

- Ionizing radiation is known to damage genes. About half the average person's exposure to ionizing radiation comes from diagnostic x-rays and medical radiation treatments. Decline all routine x-rays, and allow only those x-rays that are absolutely necessary. It is paradoxical that physicians, who put so much stock in the genetic origins of disease, inflict massive genetic damage with radiation.

- Toxins that damage genes include man-made industrial chemicals, prescription drugs, tobacco, chemical residues such as PCBs and dioxins in meat and dairy products, fluoride, and heavy metals such as mercury and lead. Foods heated to high temperatures or blackened (as in barbecuing) contain chemicals capable of causing gene mutations and cancer.

- While it doesn't cause mutations, nonionizing radiation also has genetic repercussions. As a general rule, avoid close proximity or prolonged exposure to all types of electrical devices, electrical boxes, transformers, cell phones, cell phone towers, and high-voltage power lines.

Support DNA Repair

Inherited genes are not the cause of our epidemic of cancer and premature aging and chronic disease; it is the damage we are doing to our genes. Life in the twenty-first century is damaging genes and creating mutations in unprecedented ways and at an alarming rate. Fortunately, genetic damage can be repaired. In addition to avoiding damaging our genes, we also must provide them with the raw materials (nutrients) they need to repair themselves.

Genes get damaged all the time, which is why we have DNA repair systems. However, due to our poor diets and our massive exposure to toxins and radiation, our DNA repair systems are having a difficult time keeping up with the damage. Critical DNA repairs are not getting done, and sometimes the genetic damage even disables the repair machinery.

If DNA is damaged and not repaired before the cell divides to form a new cell, the damage becomes permanent and shows up in all the new cells. The effects of this can range from minor to devastating, as the damage is cumulative. If genetic mutations take place in a sex cell, there is a 50/50 chance of passing these on to future generations. Damaged cells and genes can lead to premature aging and a variety of disease conditions including fatigue, poor resistance to infections, psychological stress, social maladjustment, and cancer.

Certain nutrients are known to support the DNA repair process. These include vitamins B3, B6, and B12; folate; zinc; and L-carnitine. Most Americans are deficient in these nutrients. According to the USDA, 73 percent of Americans are deficient in zinc, 40 percent are deficient in B12, and 80 percent are deficient in B6. Augmenting your diet with high-quality supplements is essential. Unless you supply the nutrients the body needs to make DNA repairs, the job will go undone, and genetic mutations will result.

Epigenetic Changes Give
Wrong Instructions to Healthy Genes

A mutation is a permanent change in a gene's coding. An epigenetic change, due to environmental factors, alters the function of normal, undamaged genes without changing the coding itself. However, epigenetic changes are becoming a big problem. Environmental pollutants can cause aging and disease through epigenetic changes, and worse, there is evidence that, like mutations, epigenetic changes can be passed on to future generations—one more reason to make the effort to avoid exposing yourself to environmental toxins and to do what is necessary to reduce your existing toxic load.

In addition to toxins, poor nutrition causes epigenetic changes. A mother's malnutrition can permanently alter the expression of genes in her offspring without changing the genes themselves. This is a major factor in the poor health of our current generation of children. Part of our cancer epidemic results from our consumption of nutritionally deficient processed foods over several generations; even the nutrition of your grandparents can affect how your genes express and your susceptibility to disease. The toxins we are exposed to and what we eat have far-reaching consequences beyond the damage they do to us and our own children. The future of the species is being affected.

Conclusion

- Despite popular belief, when it comes to disease, we control our genes; our genes do not control us. Most genes are DNA codes that can be expressed in thousands of different ways with thousands of different biological outcomes, and they respond to instructions we give them. We instruct our genes through the cellular environments we create with our lifestyle choices.

- A good diet, exercise, meditation, sunlight, fresh air, adequate sleep, systemic alkalinity, a normal sodium/potassium balance, limiting toxic exposures, detoxification, hormonal balance, and a positive attitude create an optimal cellular environment for genetic expression.

- Genes get damaged and repaired all the time. Ideally, repair keeps pace with damage. When it does not, mutations occur. Mutations introduce chaos into biological systems, leading to cancer and other types of disease. Another kind of damage, epigenetic change, alters gene function without altering the DNA code. These come from environmental chemicals and poor nutrition interacting with genes and interfering with their normal expression. Mutated genes and epigenetic changes can both be passed down through generations.

- Life in the twenty-first century is damaging our genes and creating mutations in unprecedented ways and at an alarming rate. You can stop much of this damage by avoiding toxins, as well as ionizing and nonionizing radiation wherever possible.

- Support DNA repair by optimizing your nutrient intake, especially vitamins B3, B6, and B12; folate; zinc; and L-carnitine. Most Americans are deficient in one or more of these nutrients.

YOUR MAINTENANCE LIST
FOR THE GENETIC PATHWAY:

Energy Production

Genes responsible for energy production must be protected from mutations and epigenetic changes.

Inflammation

Get adequate sleep. Sleep deficits affect genes that control inflammation.

Acid/Alkaline Balance

Keep your pH balanced. Cellular pH affects how genes express.

Digestive Health

Mutations and epigenetic changes can affect critical gene pathways in the gut, affecting nutrient uptake and transport into the body.

Hormonal Balance

Keep your hormones balanced. They are genetic switches.

Minimize stress. Stress hormones can change gene expression for the worse.

Get adequate sleep. Sleep helps to regulate hormones.

Sugar unbalances hormones.

Meat and dairy contain hormones that unbalance your hormones.

Platelet Stickiness

Genes responsible for platelet stickiness must be protected from mutations and epigenetic changes.

Fat Storage

Exercise regularly, because genes that control obesity are changed for the better.

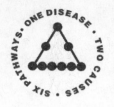

ELEVEN

Death by Medicine

*The cause of most disease is in the
poisonous drugs physicians superstitiously
give in order to effect a cure.*

—Charles E. Page, M.D.

*Doctors give drugs of which they know little,
into bodies, of which they know less, for diseases
of which they know nothing at all.*

—Voltaire

*One of the first duties of the physician is to
educate the masses not to take medicine.*

—Sir William Osler, M.D.

C onventional (allopathic) medicine is one of the biggest
misadventures in history. Every nation practicing conventional medicine is facing bankruptcy. Conventional medicine

is costly, produces few benefits, and keeps people sick. Best described as plausible pseudo-science, it is a major cause of disease and the leading cause of death in the United States. This chapter helps you to use the best that medicine has to offer while protecting yourself from its many errors.

Most of conventional medicine is based on the use of prescription drugs. But nobody is sick because of a drug deficiency! People are sick because they are deficient in nutrients and loaded with toxins. They have stressed their bodies in numerous ways, and have disabled vital defense and repair mechanisms. Drugs cause disease, disability, and death because they are toxins that poison the body and create nutrient deficiencies.

Most of the remainder of conventional medicine is based on surgery. How did we ever come to believe that removing body parts helps sick people? To be in optimum health, we need all our organs. If a body part appears to be misbehaving, we should restore its cells to normal function—not remove it. Removing body parts creates new deficiencies and toxicities, resulting in more disease.

Modern medicine works well for trauma care and crisis intervention, but beyond that it is ineffective and dangerous. If you desire true health, you must protect yourself from most of conventional medicine. The Medical Pathway is about replacing drugs and surgery with safe alternatives and shunning all unnecessary medical procedures, including screening, diagnostics, vaccinations, and medical and dental x-rays.

Conventional Medicine Does More Harm than Good

Have you noticed that people on prescription drugs age faster? This happens because drugs interfere with the normal functioning of your cells, which makes you sick. Conventional medicine tries to suppress symptoms by assaulting the body with toxic chemicals, but suppressing symptoms does nothing to cure your disease.

The drug approach is doomed to failure because it interferes with normal cell chemistry and makes you sicker. When drugs fail, surgery is often recommended. But surgery only further escalates the violence against your body. Modern medical treatments do damage along every one of the Six Pathways:

- *Nutrition Pathway.* Many drugs damage the gastrointestinal tract, impairing the ability to absorb nutrients. Others strip the body of nutrients. Taking drugs for extended periods produces deficiencies that age your body and vastly increase your risk of every disease.

- *Toxin Pathway.* The definition of a poison is "a substance that retards a reaction or destroys or inhibits a catalyst." This is precisely what prescription drugs do—they are poisons.

- *Mental Pathway.* Just being "diagnosed" with a "serious illness" is a shock from which some people never recover. When, on top of that, doctors estimate how long a patient will live, or predict that he will never walk or see again, they can demoralize the patient and create a self-fulfilling prophecy. Most doctors don't have time to listen to the patient; they discourage him from tuning in to his own body and offer little or no moral support on the path of recovery and healing.

- *Physical Pathway.* Surgery, x-rays, radiation, and other medical procedures physically damage the body and ultimately cause malfunction and disease.

- *Genetic Pathway.* Certain drugs and ionizing radiation, such as x-rays, are known to cause genetic damage. Genetic mutations can cause premature aging, cancer, and other diseases, and may be passed on to future generations.

Why You Shouldn't Always Trust Your Doctor

Although most physicians go into their profession with a genuine desire to help the sick and relieve pain and suffering, they get caught up in an outmoded, unscientific paradigm. They too become victims of a dysfunctional system that causes unnecessary suffering and death to millions.

Today's medical school education is, for the most part, controlled by drug companies, whose interest is to sell more drugs. Medical students learn virtually nothing about health or nutrition, the treatments taught have little basis in science, and they are oblivious to how dangerous these treatments are. Students are not trained to look for the underlying causes of illness but to prescribe toxic chemicals that mask symptoms of disease.

One of the most important scientific discoveries of the twentieth century was *biochemical individuality*: every human being is biologically unique and has unique nutritional requirements. Yet medicine ignores this discovery and treats everyone the same, using one-size-fits-all protocols.

Oxford University professor Sir George Pickering, M.D., one of the world's most respected experts in medical education, said in a 1971 *British Medical Journal*, "Medical education in the U.S. is, to a large extent, worship at the improbable shrine of worthless knowledge. We produce 'scientific illiterates' . . . who are not scientific in their approach to clinical questions or new technologies."

Students are not encouraged to question the current standard of care—quite the opposite. A physician can lose their license by failing to follow "prevailing standards of practice" in their community. If they don't, they can lose their licenses, even if no patient has been harmed, no patient has complained, and even if the condition of the patients has actually improved.

Conventional Medicine Is Bad Science

Modern medicine dazzles the eye and intrigues the mind with an ever-growing array of sophisticated tools and technologies. But apart from emergency care, it is remarkably ineffective. While our physicians employ lots of fancy and expensive gadgets, their level of thinking is still stuck in the seventeenth century. In 1960, health care cost 4.5 percent of the GDP. In 2010, it cost 17.4 percent, an almost 400 percent increase. Yet despite enormous increases in costs, there has been little improvement in health. Chronic disease rages out of control, and the great American health hoax continues.

Modern medicine long ago parted ways with modern science and continues to rely on a seventeenth-century understanding of the human body. In 1687 Isaac Newton's discovery of the laws of motion led to a "mechanistic" view of the universe, in which the human body was seen as a machine with parts that could be individually understood and adjusted, like a clock.

In the early twentieth century, Albert Einstein changed the Newtonian view of the world by proving that matter and energy are interchangeable. Einstein created a new paradigm in which human beings are regarded as networks of complex energy systems. But our physicians are still stuck in the seventeenth-century Newtonian model, thinking that we operate like a mechanical clock. In truth, we function more like an iPad. We are programmed, battery-operated electronic devices, and each cell contains electronic components including diodes and microprocessors. Without a correct understanding of the nature of the human body, medical practice is doomed to failure.

Most people believe that their doctors' treatments use the latest science. Not so! Several studies, including one by the U.S. Office of Technology Assessment, concluded that only 10 to 15 percent of conventional medical treatment has any basis in science. In this small area, primarily crisis intervention and trauma care, medicine excels. The other 85 to 90 percent of medical practice has never been proven by scientific method to be safe or effective. A 2011 study in the *Archives of Internal Medicine* found that even when doctors follow existing medical guidelines to the letter, 86 percent of the time they are using treatments that have little or no scientific support.

Doctors follow existing guidelines, trusting that the medical authorities who sit on guideline-drafting panels know what they're doing. They don't. Guidelines are based more on their assumptions and opinions, usually heavily influenced by the interests of the pharmaceutical industry.

There is little or no evidence that many widely used treatments and procedures actually work better than cheaper and safer alternatives, or even better than placebos. In general, conventional medicine's treatments don't work. For example, if you have cancer in more than one place, and most people do by the time they are diagnosed, your chance of being alive after five years is close to zero if you follow your doctor's advice.

Nicholas Gonzales, M.D., a prominent cancer specialist, had this to say: "The way you have to look at medicine is not as a scientific profession, but rather a religious profession. It has its irrational beliefs. It has its own special language. It has its tools, it has its rituals. The fact that they don't make us better is ignored."

Physicians get no training in scientifically advanced molecular medicine, which emphasizes cellular and molecular interventions with nontoxic nutrients. Most have no idea how to read, interpret, and understand a scientific paper. Meanwhile, the "medical literature," increasingly influenced by drug company money, is more and more untrustworthy. This is bad science, which is why the eminent scientist Linus Pauling called most cancer research "a fraud."

The situation is so serious that in 2001 the prestigious Institute of Medicine of the National Academy of Sciences issued a report, *Crossing the Quality Chasm*, which concluded, "Between the health care we now have and the health care we could have lies not just a gap but a chasm." The report also said,

> *The nation's health care delivery system has fallen short in its ability to translate knowledge into practice and to apply new technology safely and appropriately.... If the system cannot consistently deliver today's science and technology, it is even less prepared to respond to the extraordinary advances that surely will emerge during the coming decades.*

Conventional medicine waits for disease to happen. Then it attempts to suppress the symptoms with toxic drugs and invasive surgery, doing enormous, often irreparable—even fatal—damage to the body. This irrational approach not only runs up the costs, it makes your disease chronic, leaves you sicker than when you started, and may even kill you. This hopelessly outdated system needs to be replaced with science-based medicine.

Conventional Medicine Is a Business

The disease industry is dependent on millions of people getting sick and, more important, staying sick. It has little economic incentive to prevent or cure disease. It is designed to perpetuate the management of symptoms and to keep the money flowing.

Forbes magazine estimates U.S. national healthcare expenditures for 2014 at $3.8 trillion. Three out of four of these dollars (roughly $2.8 trillion) are spent treating entirely preventable chronic conditions. It costs a lot more to fix something after it is broken than to prevent it from breaking in the first place. Yet conventional medicine makes almost no attempt to prevent disease, and its treatments do far more harm than good.

Conventional Medicine Is the Leading Cause of Death

From medical errors to adverse drug reactions to unnecessary procedures, conventional medicine is literally killing us, and the numbers are right there in the medical statistics. A number of analyses—including those in Dr. Carolyn Dean's 2005 book, *Death by Modern Medicine*; Gary Null's 2010 book, *Death by Medicine*; the 1991 *Harvard Medical Practice Study*; the 1994 *Journal of the American Medical Association* article, "Error in Medicine"; and others—have shown that conventional medicine causes more harm than good.

The authors of the above analyses took statistics right from the most respected medical and scientific journals and investigative reports by the Institute of Medicine. They have clearly demonstrated that *medical intervention is the leading cause of death in the United States*, killing more than 1 million people per year. According to the 2011 *Health-Grades Hospital Quality and Clinical Excellence Study*, the incidence rate of medical harm is now over 40,000 harmful/lethal errors daily. The Nutrition Institute of America in its October 2003 report, *Death by Medicine*, concluded, "Our estimated 10-year total of 7.8 million iatrogenic [doctor-induced] deaths is more than all the casualties from all the wars fought by the U.S. throughout its entire history." Amazing, isn't it? In just one ten-year period, doctors killed more people than all of our wars combined. Given these statistics, it is ironic that while conventional medicine and prescription drugs are killing people by the millions, the focus of government regulators is on banning and restricting the use of vitamins that prevent and cure disease and kill no one.

How does conventional medicine get away with killing millions of people? The combination of powerful business interests and relentless brainwashing through the medical establishment and mass media has created a culture where convention prevails over science and common sense. How many people religiously observe their annual flu shots and their mammograms? Yet these, along with hundreds of other routine medical procedures, have been shown to offer little value while causing considerable harm.

Screening Doesn't Prevent Anything

The only way to prevent disease is to supply your cells with the nutrients they need and protect them from toxins and physical harm. The disease industry aggressively promotes screening for cancer and other diseases. *But screening does not prevent anything.* What it offers is a trade-off between the possible risk of a late diagnosis and the very real and tangible harm of an invasive medical procedure.

Colonoscopy

Since television journalist Katie Couric's televised colonoscopy in 2000, colorectal cancer screening rates have soared. The American Cancer Society recommends that, starting at age fifty, everyone get a colonoscopy every ten years, or a CT colonography (virtual colonoscopy) every five years. According to the CDC, 59 percent of the U.S. population between the ages of fifty and seventy-five follow these guidelines. Yet everyone can take simple steps to virtually eliminate the risk of getting colon cancer. Recall from chapter 3 that never browning your meat brings down your odds of getting colon cancer; consuming mostly whole plant-based foods brings the risk of any cancer close to zero. On the other hand, a colonoscopy has a number of well-known risks and side effects:

- *Disruption of intestinal flora.* Synthetic laxatives and enemas routinely prescribed to clean out the intestines before a colonoscopy damage gut bacteria. This can result in constipation, irritable bowel syndrome, diverticulitis, ulcerative colitis, and Crohn's disease, which raise the risk of colon cancer.

- *Postinterventional complications.* Serious complications, such as colon perforation, occur in five out of every 1,000 colonoscopies. The risks of delayed bleeding, infection, and ulceration are even higher, but they rarely get reported. Biopsy or polyp removal increases the risk of complications.

- *Increased risk of deferred strokes, heart attacks, and pulmonary embolisms.* Blood clotting is a common side effect of anesthesia, particularly among patients with diabetes or heart disease. These blood clots may cause a deadly pulmonary embolism, stroke, or heart attack weeks after the colonoscopy.

- *Infections.* Any medical procedure performed under anesthesia raises your risk for an infectious disease, like pneumonia.

- *False negatives.* According to multiple studies, doctors miss from 15 to 27 percent of polyps, including 6 percent of large tumors. Some doctors do so many procedures in one day, and rush through the colon exam so fast, they miss cancer in full bloom.

According to the American College of Gastroenterology, virtual colonoscopies miss 27 percent of colorectal lesions, including precancerous colon polyps and actual cancerous tumors. And if the radiologist finds a polyp or two, you'll need to undergo a regular colonoscopy anyway to remove them. False positive readings are also common. Plus, abdominal CT scans expose you to a massive dose of cancer-causing radiation.

Bottom line: Colonoscopies, actual and virtual, are dangerous medical procedures that expose you to physical harm, toxic drugs, and disruption of vital processes in the body, while doing nothing to lower your risk of colon cancer. In fact, they increase your risk of cancer. If you are serious about preventing colon cancer and staying biologically young, change your diet and stay away from CT scanners and other unnecessary medical tests.

Diagnostic X-Rays

X-rays cause cancer. John Gofman, M.D., Ph.D., both a medical doctor and a nuclear physicist, was one of the world's leading experts on radiation damage. His groundbreaking book, *Radiation from Medical Procedures in the Pathogenesis of Cancer and Ischemic Heart Disease*, was published in 1999. According to Gofman, there is no "safe" level of radiation. Each additional exposure to radiation increases your risk of getting cancer.

Whether from CT scans or chest x-rays, Americans today are exposed to seven times more radiation from diagnostic x-rays than they were in 1980. Most of the average person's lifetime radiation exposure comes from diagnostic x-rays, yet there is no medical justification for as much as 90 percent of them, including routine x-rays like mammograms.

Mammograms expose your body to radiation that can be 1,000 times greater than a chest x-ray. Gofman's three decades of research into the effects of low-dose radiation on humans indicated that medical x-rays play an essential role in about 75 percent of all breast cancers. Cancer statistics show that breast cancer has increased since the introduction of mammographic screening in 1983. A 1995 study on mammograms in the *Lancet* concluded, "The benefit is marginal, the harm caused is substantial, and the costs incurred are enormous." A growing body of new research has come to this same conclusion. Mammograms save few lives and lead to unnecessary, expensive, and dangerous treatments. Unfortunately, a growing number of doctors are rated and compensated on the percentage of their patients who are up-to-date on their screenings.

Mammography also compresses the breasts (often painfully), which could cause the spread of any existing malignant cells. Mammograms have a high rate of false positives. About 5 percent of mammograms suggest further testing; over 90 percent of those are false positives. This results in unnecessary expense, emotional trauma, needless biopsies, and other unnecessary surgical procedures. Mammograms also produce a high rate of false negatives. According to the National Cancer Institute, for women in the forty to forty-nine age group, the rate of missed tumors is 40 percent! Mammograms don't save lives. Research shows that adding an annual mammogram to a careful physical examination of the breasts does not improve breast cancer survival rates.

Fortunately, there is a better way—a safe, accurate, and inexpensive diagnostic test called a thermogram. Thermography measures the temperature of the breast, without mechanical pressure or ionizing radiation. It can detect breast cancer as much as ten years earlier than a mammogram. A growing tumor requires its own blood supply. The increased blood flow makes that area warmer than the surrounding tissue. This temperature differential can be accurately measured, with no false negatives and few false positives, without any danger or discomfort to the patient.

Another abuse of x-rays is the widespread use of computed tomography (CT) scans. Originally known as computed axial tomography (CAT) scans, the use of these x-ray scanners has increased dramatically over the last couple of decades. An estimated 75 million–plus scans are now being performed in the United States annually. CT scans can image the entire human body within seconds, producing high-definition images that provide physicians with an incredibly detailed view of the organs and tissues deep within us.

While CT scans can be beneficial for certain situations, like serious injury from multiple traumas, overuse of these devices is rampant. Healthy people are being exposed to excessive, cancer-causing radiation for clinically dubious screening purposes.

A CT coronary artery angiogram can deliver the same amount of radiation as 310 chest x-rays. Two studies published in the 2009 *Archives of Internal Medicine* found enormous variations in the amount of radiation being delivered by different CT imaging facilities. Thirteen-fold variations have been found between the highest and lowest doses for the same type of scan. Some people received such grossly excessive radiation doses that their hair began falling out. The risk of developing cancer is proportional to the dose of radiation received, and CT scans deliver a lot. These researchers estimated that the CT scans done in 2007 alone will result in approximately 29,000 future cases of cancer caused directly by the scans. This conservative estimate does not account for those with nutritional deficiencies or a poorly functioning DNA repair system, who will be especially vulnerable to the ill effects of radiation.

Biopsy

Needle biopsies are widely used and accepted as a safe procedure for diagnosing cancer. But they are not safe. As early as 1940, medical experts warned that needle biopsies could cause cancer cells to break away from a tumor and spread to other parts of the body. A 2007 study in the *British Medical Journal* confirmed this suspicion. *If you have a needle biopsy, you are 50 percent more likely to have your cancer spread.* The body tries to wall off tumors. When you poke a hole in this protective capsule, cancer cells can spill out directly into the bloodstream or lymphatic system and spread throughout the body.

Prescription Drugs Create Disease

Prescription drugs are one of our leading causes of disease—a major contributor to our chronic disease epidemic—and the third-leading cause of death in the United States. Everyone wants a magic pill to cure disease, but there is no such thing. The risk of taking these drugs far exceeds their potential benefits.

By making the body both deficient and toxic, prescription drugs damage the body's overall resistance to disease. Properly prescribed prescription drugs hospitalize about 4.5 million people and kill an estimated 500,000 or more every year. In addition, prescription drugs decrease the quality of life for tens of millions. Drugs are toxic to mitochondria and inhibit energy production. Most prescription drugs, including antibiotics, have an acidic effect on the body. Drugs even upset fat storage control and cause weight gain, especially birth control, antidepressant, and diabetes drugs.

Americans Are Overmedicated

Every month about 130 million Americans swallow, inject, inhale, infuse, spray, and pat on prescribed medications, according to the CDC. America uses more medicine per person than any other country in the world. According to pharmaceutical consulting company IMS Health, the number of prescriptions has grown by two-thirds over the past decade to 3.5 billion yearly.

"We are taking way too many drugs for dubious or exaggerated ailments," says Dr. Marcia Angell, former editor of the *New England Journal of Medicine* and author of *The Truth About the Drug Companies*. "What the drug companies are doing now is promoting drugs for long-term use to essentially healthy people. Why? Because it's the biggest market."

Drug makers, doctors, and patients' have all been quick to medicate some conditions once accepted simply as part of the human condition. Potent drugs, like beta-blockers, are even being used as "prophylactic measures" in people having no complaints at all.

The average person thinks that they need their drugs to lower their blood pressure, lower their cholesterol, treat their depression, and so on. In truth, virtually no one *needs* a drug. It is difficult to think of a prescription drug for which there is not an alternative treatment that is safer, less expensive, and more effective. Every time independent researchers take a serious look at a prescription drug, they find it is dangerous. Find an alternative doctor who will help you get well, and not use you, knowingly or unknowingly, to enrich the medical/pharmaceutical establishment.

Remember, no drug, no matter how common, is safe. In fact, quite the opposite is true. By widely promoting dangerous disease-causing drugs, the industry creates the impression they must be safe, effective, and worth the cost, and hides the enormous damage they do. Let's have a look at some of the most common medications you should stop taking as soon as possible.

Birth Control Pills

Birth control pills seriously disrupt your body's hormonal balance and cause every kind of disease from depression to cancer. A 1991 study in the *Journal of the National Cancer Institute* found that women who take birth control pills for five years or more increase their risk of getting liver cancer by 550 percent over those who have never taken them.

Birth control pills cause numerous other problems, including mood swings, vitamin deficiencies, blood clots and stroke, weight gain, and multiple sclerosis. These dangerous drugs also disrupt the normal balance of the bacteria in your gut and cause bowel disorders such as Crohn's disease.

TNF Blockers

Tumor necrosis factor (TNF) blockers are used to treat inflammatory and autoimmune diseases such as Crohn's disease and rheumatoid arthritis. The FDA has ordered manufacturers to include a "black box warning" about an increased risk of cancer in children and adolescents. This is the most severe warning that the FDA can place on a product without withdrawing it from the market. In response to numerous reports of children developing cancer while taking these drugs, the FDA concluded in 2009 that "there is an increased risk of lymphoma and other cancers associated with the use of these drugs in children and adolescents." It would be foolhardy not to assume they are also risky for adults. Another problem with TNF blockers is that they depress immunity, opening the door to serious infections such as tuberculosis.

Antibiotics

Most people think of antibiotics as one of conventional medicine's greatest triumphs. In fact, they are one of the greatest medical blunders in history. Virtually everyone who has ever taken these dangerous and unnecessary drugs has suffered permanent damage to their health. There are safer ways to treat infections. Once you have taken an antibiotic, the only real options are to never take another, and try to compensate for the prior damage as best you can with a high-fiber diet and high-quality probiotics.

The purpose of antibiotics is to treat infections by killing bacteria. However, they also destroy the beneficial bacteria in your gut—and that's the problem. Recall from chapter 4 that the assortment of gut flora in each of us is as unique as a fingerprint. Your unique flora helps to support your unique biochemistry. Taking even one course of antibiotics can destroy this uniqueness. Once destroyed, you cannot reconstitute it.

Once this vital "organ" is permanently damaged, your health is compromised, and there will be lasting weakness where there was once strength. Studies show that women who have taken antibiotics have compromised flora and produce children with compromised flora; the damage is being passed on to the unborn and to future generations.

A properly functioning intestinal tract is one of your first lines of defense against disease, and declining levels of friendly intestinal bacteria contribute to every imaginable disease from the common cold to asthma, allergies, Crohn's disease, and autoimmune syndromes. The brain and nervous system are damaged, and cancer is promoted.

About 80 percent of our immune system is located in the intestines. As such, abnormal gut bacteria depress immunity and the body's ability to repair. Stripping your gut of its natural balance of healthy bacteria promotes an overgrowth of harmful microorganisms such as parasites, mycoplasma, fungi, yeasts like candida, and hostile bacteria such as Pseudomonas, Clostridium, and Klebsiella. Once this happens, your immunity is severely impaired. The harmful microorganisms produce many toxins. These toxins affect endocrine glands, causing hypothyroidism and adrenal insufficiency; they also produce numerous cognitive and neurological problems similar to multiple sclerosis and amyotrophic lateral sclerosis. A 2012 study in the *FASEB Journal* suggests that harmful bacteria in the intestines cause heart attacks, while maintaining healthy intestinal flora may help reduce heart attack risk. As mentioned in chapter 4, studies show that the more times you take an antibiotic, the higher your risk of developing cancer. Gerald Weissmann, M.D., editor in chief of the *FASEB Journal*, said, "We may soon evaluate our body's susceptibility to disease by looking at the microbes that inhabit the gut."

Another harmful effect of the rampant abuse of antibiotics is the creation of bacteria strains that are antibiotic-resistant. They cause illnesses that are difficult, if not impossible, to treat with standard procedures. Threatening a global pandemic, these deadly superbugs are ravaging our hospitals and rapidly moving out into the general population. About half of all our hospital rooms are now infected, killing at least 50,000 people per year in the United States alone. Infections caught in hospitals are now the fourth-leading cause of death. Due to widespread use of antibiotics in agriculture, antibiotic-resistant bacteria are now common in the meat aisles of our supermarkets. With startlingly high percentages of store-bought meat samples being contaminated with antibiotic-resistant superbugs, these meat products have become a direct source of foodborne illness, posing special dangers to young children, pregnant women, and the elderly.

Heavy metal toxicity is now epidemic, and the bioaccumulation of mercury, lead, and other metals is making us sick. One reason this is happening is because antibiotics destroy and alter gut bacteria that help the body to rid itself of heavy metals. We are accumulating more because we are excreting less.

Good health begins in the intestinal tract. With the exception of oxygen, nutrients enter the body through the intestines. If food is not properly broken down, it will ferment and putrefy in the gut, producing powerful toxins. Once food is properly digested, nutrients from the food must be absorbed through the intestinal walls into the bloodstream. Good bacteria facilitate this absorption, while damage done to gut tissue by harmful flora impedes it. Thus, destruction of helpful bacteria results in deficiency and toxicity—the two causes of all disease.

Food allergies, immunodeficiency syndromes, and a variety of intestinal disorders can result from altered flora. Damage done by antibiotics has led to an epidemic of digestive difficulties, resulting in an enormous quantity of over-the-counter digestive aids being sold every year. Sadly, most doctors are unaware that the antibiotics they themselves prescribed have caused their patients' digestive problems. Antibiotics can decimate populations of lactobacilli. Lactobacilli assist in the production of digestive enzymes and they help increase the absorption of nutrients such as B vitamins, calcium, and essential fatty acids.

Much smaller than human cells, there are more bacteria living in our intestines than we have cells in our body. Gut bacteria degrade toxins and produce vitamins. They perform so many important functions that they are comparable to a body organ, like the heart or lungs. By taking antibiotics even once can cripple this organ permanently. Taking antibiotics often, or for extended periods, is certain to cause lifelong health problems. Eating a high-fiber diet and taking high-quality probiotic supplements, or including raw, live-culture sauerkraut or kimchi in your diet, are your best choices for helping to cope with this damage.

Even the CDC estimates that half of all antibiotic use is unnecessary, but in truth, there is no need for antibiotics at all. Effective, natural, and much safer ways are available to prevent and cure infections. Immune-enhancing nutrients such as vitamins A, C, D, and E; selenium, zinc, and quercitin; and natural antibiotics like wild oregano, liquid Kyolic, and olive leaf extract will take care of most infections. The right amount of vitamin C will stop almost any infection. Difficult infections can be resolved with intravenous vitamin C and other blood treatments such as ultraviolet light or ozone. Hyperbaric oxygen can be helpful, and there are even resonant frequency methods such as a Rife machine.

Statin Drugs

Statins, prescribed to lower cholesterol, are useless and dangerous. There is no scientific evidence that they lower your risk of heart attack or death. They lower cholesterol artificially by poisoning your entire body, causing incalculable harm and even death. Yet half of all men and a third of all women ages sixty-five to seventy-four are on statins.

Cholesterol is not the problem. Cholesterol is essential to human life, a building block for cell membranes and many hormones. Inflammation is the problem. Inflammation oxidizes cholesterol, and causes heart disease. Whether your cholesterol is high or low doesn't matter: when cholesterol oxidizes, you get the same damaging result, which is why half of all heart attacks occur in people with perfectly normal cholesterol levels. There are as many heart attacks in people with cholesterol levels under 200 as in those whose levels are over 300. In Crete, the home of the healthy Mediterranean diet, there are virtually no heart attacks despite average cholesterol levels well over 200. The French have the highest average cholesterol in Europe, around 250, but the lowest incidence of heart disease and half the heart attacks we have here in the United States. The solution is to prevent inflammation, not to lower cholesterol.

Statins damage the liver. They damage the heart muscle. By depleting CoQ10, statins cause congestive heart failure, which has increased alarmingly since their introduction. They increase the risk of cancer. Statins damage the brain, causing impaired memory, amnesia, confusion, disorientation, and neuropathies. Other problems caused by statins include muscle pain and weakness; stroke; cataracts; pancreatitis; respiratory and urinary problems; sleep disorders; sexual dysfunction; psychological problems like depression, anxiety, hostility, and homicidal impulses; kidney failure; plantar fasciitis; stomach ulcers; insomnia; dizziness; tremors; loss of libido; impotence; joint pain; high blood sugar; vertigo; hepatitis; and dry, "crocodile" skin. Statins have also been associated with Parkinson's, Alzheimer's, and amyotrophic lateral sclerosis (ALS; Lou Gehrig's disease).

Many side effects don't occur until weeks and sometimes years after commencing the drug. Cancer is one long-term side effect that may be missed, because most human studies with statins are time-limited. Statins have caused cancer in animals in multiple studies, and in one human study reported in a 1996 issue of the *New England Journal of Medicine*, breast cancer rates went up 1,500 percent among statin users.

Oxidized cholesterol is the real culprit in cardiovascular disease, and it can be avoided by eating an anti-inflammatory diet, taking antioxidant supplements, getting sugar out of your life, and exercising regularly. Supplement with antioxidants like coenzyme Q10, vitamins C and E, and omega-3 fatty acids, which are far more effective than statins in reducing both heart disease and all-cause mortality.

Baby Aspirin for Blood Clots

Many physicians prescribe a daily baby aspirin to reduce the chances of heart attack or stroke. This is a big mistake. The body knows how to prevent unwanted clots, strokes, and heart attacks. Your job is to support the body, not try to force the issue with toxic drugs. Most people have no idea how dangerous even a baby aspirin can be. Aspirin acts as a blood thinner, which can lead to gastrointestinal bleeding and brain hemorrhage. In fact, you are at increased risk for bruising and bleeding for two days after taking a single baby aspirin. Aspirin can lower kidney efficiency, promoting congestive heart failure. It can even trigger asthma in some individuals.

The winning solution is to give the body what it needs to prevent blood clots. Keep your platelets unsticky by eating a good diet and avoiding the Bad Four. Supplement with vitamins C and E, B12, B complex, folate, magnesium, beta-carotene, quercitin, olive oil, and essential fatty acids. These will be far safer and more effective than any drug.

Vaccines

Another of conventional medicine's historic fiascos is vaccinations. Vaccines are ineffective and dangerous. Unlike other drugs, which undergo basic testing prior to approval and recommendation, vaccines do not have to be proven safe or effective before hitting the market. While there is no scientific evidence that immunizations prevent disease, there is plenty of evidence that they are not safe. No vaccine has ever been scientifically proven in double-blind, placebo-controlled studies to be effective; the existing evidence indicates they are only marginally effective or not effective at all.

There is a lack of scientific understanding of what vaccines do and how they interact with the body. Despite this ignorance, they are widely used and cause serious harm. The typical child gets forty-eight doses of fourteen vaccines by six years of age, and sixty-nine doses of sixteen vaccines by age eighteen. These vaccines weaken the immune system and damage the brain. Unvaccinated children are healthier, less likely to get sick, and more intelligent.

The enormous increase in autism rates, now one in fifty children, coincides with the sharp increase in vaccination schedules. Infant monkeys given standard doses of childhood vaccines develop autism, and the mechanism by which this happens is now understood.

A 2011 study in *Human and Experimental Toxicology* found a correlation between a nation's vaccination rates and its infant mortality rate. The United States is the most vaccinated country in the world, and despite the many other factors that tend to lower our infant mortality, thirty-three nations have better infant mortality rates. Researchers are now attributing the epidemics of asthma, autoimmune disease, cerebral palsy, infantile convulsions, sudden infant death syndrome, and even cancer to vaccinations.

No vaccine has ever been tested to see if it is carcinogenic, yet we inject these dangerous toxic concoctions into our children. After accidents, cancer has become the leading cause of death for our young people. Vaccines contain mercury compounds, aluminum, and formaldehyde, substances that are known to cause cancer. Vaccines also contain viruses, and certain viruses are known to cause cancer. For example, a monkey virus, SV40, found in polio vaccine has been proven to cause cancer in humans. Researchers believe that SV40 is responsible for an epidemic of lung, brain, bone, and lymphatic cancers. Two independent studies published in *Lancet* in 2002 estimated that up to half of the 55,000 annual cases of non-Hodgkin's lymphoma can be attributed to polio vaccine received decades ago. In addition, vaccines drive cancer by depressing immunity.

In exchange for all this damage, vaccines offer little if any protection. In nearly every outbreak of infectious disease, the majority of the children affected are those who have been vaccinated against the organism. In 2010 the largest outbreak of whooping cough in the last half century occurred in California. Over 80 percent of the cases occurred in people who were fully vaccinated, and those who were vaccinated were more likely to get the disease than the unvaccinated. Further, the use of these vaccines has produced a new strain of whooping cough that is far more dangerous. Research shows that people who have flu shots are more likely to be infected by the flu. Further, people who get flu shots five years in a row increase their risk of Alzheimer's disease by 1,000 percent.

The dramatic decline of infectious diseases such as smallpox, diphtheria, and polio is often cited as proof of vaccinations' effectiveness. But the incidence of infectious disease decreased dramatically before the introduction of vaccines. In other words, vaccines get credit for something they did not do. For example, in 1950 the polio epidemic was at its height in Great Britain. By the time the polio vaccine was introduced in 1956, polio had already declined by 82 percent.

Australian researcher Viera Scheibner, Ph.D., author of the book *Vaccination*, investigated over 60,000 pages of medical literature on vaccination and found,

> *Immunizations, including those practiced on babies, not only did not prevent any infectious diseases; they caused more suffering and more deaths than has any other human activity in the entire history of medical intervention.*

Canadian physician Dr. Guylaine Lanctot, author of the bestseller *The Medical Mafia*, puts it this way:

> *The medical authorities keep lying. Vaccination has been an assault on the immune system. It actually causes a lot of illnesses. We are actually changing our genetic code through vaccination. . . . . 100 years from now we will know that the biggest crime against humanity was vaccines.*

Renowned pediatrician and author Dr. Robert Mendelsohn was equally direct in his book *Confessions of a Medical Heretic*:

> *Much of what you have been led to believe about immunization simply isn't true. . . . There is no convincing scientific evidence that mass inoculations can be credited with eliminating any childhood disease.*

Medical researcher Juan Manuel Martínez Méndez, M.D., writing in a 2004 *Townsend Letter* (a respected examiner of medical alternatives), stated,

These chronic diseases, including hay fever, asthma, cancer, and AIDS, are the result of wrong interventions upon the organism by conventional medicine . . . The immune systems of the Western population, through strong chemical drugs and repeated vaccinations, have broken down. . . . Medicine, instead of curing diseases, is actually the cause of the degeneration of the human race.

Aluminum has been added to vaccines for about ninety years in the belief that it spurs the body to produce disease-fighting antibodies. Eighteen of the thirty-six vaccines children get contain large doses of aluminum, up to forty-six times the maximum dose considered safe by regulatory agencies. Pneumonia, tetanus, and HPV shots all contain aluminum, adding to the lifetime cumulative amounts of aluminum in adults. Research has demonstrated that aluminum is an accumulative neurotoxin, even in small concentrations. It has a tendency to concentrate in the hippocampus—an area of the brain vital to crucial functions, including learning, memory, and behavior—causing neurological disorders in children and adults.

As we age, our brains become progressively more inflamed, and aluminum accelerates and magnifies that inflammation. Aluminum displaces iron from its protective proteins. This increases the level of free iron in the body and triggers intense inflammation, free radical generation, and lipid peroxidation. There is also powerful evidence that aluminum worsens the effects of other toxins, such as pesticides, herbicides, mercury, and fluoride. In essence, accumulating aluminum damages your brain. The incidence of neurological disorders like Alzheimer's, ALS, Parkinson's, and multiple sclerosis is exploding because we are bioaccumulating toxins like aluminum at an unprecedented rate.

What About Infectious Diseases

If antibiotics and vaccinations are inappropriate, how then do we deal with infectious diseases? The answer is simple: keep your immunity strong. The "bug" is not the problem. The problem is when we create a biological environment that allows the bug to grow and prosper. We create that environment by eating sugar and an overall poor diet, and with toxins, stress, lack of sleep, and other factors. Studies show that only a small percentage of those exposed to a specific virus actually get sick. Only those with the weakest immunity get sick. Studies of college students show that more students get sick during exam times because their immunity is lowered by the stress and the loss of sleep while cramming for exams. Keeping your immune system strong and healthy is paramount.

Remember, there is only one disease and only two causes of disease. When we cause cells to malfunction and lower our immunity, microorganisms can grow. When this happens, the microorganisms make us sick by causing even more deficiency, toxicity, and cellular malfunction. While infectious agents such as bacteria, viruses, fungi, and others are involved in the disease process, it is not the organism itself, but the resulting cellular malfunction that is the problem. So we are always back to one disease—cellular malfunction—with two causes, deficiency and toxicity.

We live in a sea of microorganisms. There are far more microorganisms living in and on your body than there are human cells in your body. We already have many pathogenic organisms living in our bodies, but they don't make us sick; we live in harmony with them. The "bugs" in our bodies actually support our health, and we cannot live without them. Problems occur when the natural balance between us and the microorganisms is upset, and certain bugs start to grow beyond their normal amount and others may be depressed below their normal amount. When this happens, we can be affected in different ways.

In many cases, the body is damaged because of the body's reaction to the microorganism. For example, some people with West Nile virus will develop paralysis or lapse into a coma. It used to be thought that the virus invaded the brain. Not so. The damage is done when there is an excessive immune response and the brain's own immune cells release high levels of inflammatory chemicals in reaction to the virus. These powerful chemicals have a toxic effect and damage brain cells—a similar type of excessive immune response happens with Ebola. An infection with the bacterium anthrax kills because the bacterium produces powerful toxins that poison cells, causing them to malfunction.

While most of us are familiar with acute infections, like the flu, many health problems have been linked to chronic low-level infections due to compromised immunity. How do you get an infection? Here are three factors to consider: the virulence of the organism, the number of organisms involved, and, most important, the strength of your immunity. Unfortunately, almost all of us are immune compromised to one degree or another because of nutrient deficiencies, toxic overload, stressful lifestyles, and the fact that our immune systems have been permanently damaged by vaccinations and antibiotics.

A chronic deficiency of any essential nutrient will eventually depress immunity, and most of us are deficient in nutrients essential to immune health. These include vitamins A, C, D, E and B complex. Zinc, magnesium, and selenium are also in short supply. A deficiency of omega-3 fatty acids, iron, and carotenoids also increase the likelihood of infection. For most of us, supplementation is essential. But the quality of the supplements is critical. Low-quality supplements will not do the job.

Certain toxins are known to depress immunity. These include fluoride from your water and toothpaste, as well as mercury from fish and dental fillings, pesticides, herbicides, vaccinations, and excess iron in the system. Mercury is known to dramatically increase virus production in the body, and most of us have too much mercury.

Stress, lack of sleep, low pH, antibiotics, vaccinations, surgery, radiation, and various prescription drugs all depress immunity. Sugar, stress, lack of sleep, and glutamates also depress immunity.

Supporting immune health and reducing excessive immune responses can be accomplished with good nutrition, detoxification, and supplementing with immune-supporting nutrients. Beyond vitamins and minerals, curcumin, quercitin, white tea, aged garlic extract, olive leaf extract, oregano oil, and grapeseed extract are all natural virus-fighting substances. In addition, foods that support immunity include garlic, onion, ginger, cayenne, and clove. Maintaining normal pH in your cells is very important.

As this section is being written, Ebola is epidemic in Africa and even affecting the United States. The death rate is high in Africa and people there are panicking, while Americans are justifiably concerned. Meanwhile, the inept and bloated federal bureaucracy we call the Centers for Disease Control (CDC) has bungled the job of protecting our citizens. With an annual budget of seven billion dollars, it didn't even have effective protocols in place for dealing with Ebola. It did not even recommend that exposed people restrict their travel or who travel from West Africa be restricted.

The CDC claims that restricting travel from West Africa would not be effective. That may be politically correct, but it is not medically correct. Think about it. Use common sense. If a proper travel ban had been in place, the late Thomas Duncan would not have been allowed to travel to the United States from Liberia, and we would not be having the problems we are now having. End of argument. So why is the government still allowing travel from the affected areas? The CDC is recommending airport screening, but for many valid reasons, there is no way this can ever be effective.

So what should you be doing? The answer is simple: keep your immunity strong. Pay attention to the maintenance items listed in this book, including maintaining normal pH in your cells. The best way to protect yourself is to keep your immunity strong by giving it what it needs to function optimally and keeping it free of toxins that depress it.

People are fearful because Ebola has a high mortality rate, but is there a cure for Ebola? Theoretically there is, and Ebola should be simple to cure, but no one is doing it yet. The existing literature indicates that vitamin C, in sufficient quantities, has never failed to cure any virus infection. Yet to date, there is no clinical evidence that vitamin C will cure Ebola. However, this is not because it won't cure Ebola; it's because conventional medicine isn't even trying to find out. For serious infections, in order to get serum levels high enough to do the job, intravenous administration of vitamin C is required. According to the late Dr. Robert Cathcart, a pioneer in vitamin C treatment of disease, some Ebola patients may require as much a 500 grams per day to cure the disease.

What appears to be happening to Ebola patients is that the body mounts an excessive immune response to the infection, producing a flood of inflammatory chemicals that massively damage every tissue in the body, causing the blood vessels to leak. These inflammatory chemicals use up vitamin C and cause the need for vitamin C to go sky high. The infection quickly exhausts the body's supply of vitamin C, and this deficiency causes acute scurvy, which results in further breakdown of the blood vessels. The blood vessels leak, and people die of internal hemorrhaging. All this should be possible to prevent with adequate vitamin C. As a protective measure, the Orthomolecular Medicine News Service recommends that people take at least 10 grams per day orally—I take 15 grams.

In addition to intravenous vitamin C, there are other treatments that should also be effective against Ebola including ozone treatment of the blood and Ultraviolet Blood Irradiation (UBI), also called Photoluminescence Therapy. UBI consists of removing about six ounces of blood from the patient, exposing the blood to ultraviolet light, and returning the blood to the body. The procedure takes about one hour. Decades of experience has shown that UBI is safe and can strengthen the immune system, improve overall health, and destroy fungal, viral, and bacterial growth. Unfortunately, conventional medicine is not yet even looking into ozone, UBI, or any other of these potentially life-saving treatments.

Ninety Percent of Surgeries Are Unnecessary

Surgery works very well to correct physical problems, such as those sustained in accidents, military action, sports injuries, or birth defects. But surgery does not solve disease problems. Unfortunately, most surgery in the United States is performed to address systemic diseases, like heart disease and cancer—wasting resources, while permanently damaging the patient. Surgery and anesthesia cause a variety of metabolic problems—immunosuppression for one. Surgery-induced suppression results in postoperative infections and tumor metastasis.

Surgery should never be performed unless there is no alternative. So how often is that? About 10 percent of the time. In *Confessions of a Medical Heretic*, Dr. Robert Mendelsohn says that about 90 percent of surgery is a "waste of time, money, energy, and life." He cites a study that found that most of the patients recommended for surgery did not need it, and half of them needed no medical treatment at all. In another case, a hospital oversight committee reviewed surgically removed tissues and found that most tissues being removed were healthy! That hospital had performed 262 appendectomies that year; the year following the committee's review, the number dropped to 62. In March 1997 the Physicians Committee for Responsible Medicine published a statement saying that 90 percent of hysterectomies are not justified.

Many common surgical procedures have been found to be useless. For example, in 2013 the *New England Journal of Medicine* reported that a fake surgical procedure to replace a piece of cartilage known as the meniscus in knee joints was every bit as effective as real surgery. Despite this, 700,000 of these useless procedures are done annually.

In addition to being mostly unnecessary, surgery is risky. Possibilities exist for surgical error, complications from anesthesia, and infection, not to mention the physical, mental, and emotional shock to the body. Anesthesia is dangerous. Common local anesthetics, such as lidocaine, are carcinogenic. General anesthesia significantly increases the risk of developing dementia, with the risk remaining high even years after the surgery.

Surgery Increases Inflammation

Surgery places enormous stress on the body, causing a substantial increase in the production of inflammatory chemicals, causing premature aging and lowering resistance to disease. A 2008 study published in *Experimental Gerontology* found that even minor surgery, such as removing a mole, can cause brain inflammation that contributes to disease conditions such as Alzheimer's. High levels of inflammation have been shown to stimulate the production of new blood vessels that feed tumors and also to increase cancer cell adhesion.

Heart Bypass

A heart bypass operation is a prime example of unnecessary surgery. Nortin Hadler, M.D., a professor of medicine at the University of North Carolina Medical School, said that 95 to 97 percent of coronary bypass surgeries are unnecessary—even though patients are usually told that without the surgery they will die. Bypass surgery is not benign. Patients can die during the surgery, and many are left with permanent heart rhythm problems and brain damage with memory loss. Fortunately, almost all coronary disease is preventable with diet, supplements, and exercise. Coronary disease is also reversible, as pioneers like Nathan Pritikin, Dean Ornish, M.D., and others have proven.

Another commonly overused surgical procedure is the use of small, mesh tubes called *stents* to open arteries. At hospitals where stents are the most overused, studies show that six out of ten of these procedures are inappropriate, even by existing medical standards. Good nutrition, detoxification, and exercise will clean out your arteries—surgery not required.

Hip Implants Poison Your Cells

About 250,000 Americans over age fifty undergo hip replacement surgery each year, unknowingly exposing themselves to dangerously high levels of toxic metals. A joint investigation by the BBC and the *British Medical Journal* (*BMJ*) found that toxic cobalt and chromium ions can seep into the tissues of patients with all-metal hip implants, leaving some patients with long-term disability. Studies have also shown that metal ions can damage bone and muscle, leach into the bloodstream, and spread to the lymph nodes, spleen, liver, and kidneys. There are also concerns about damage to chromosomes that can lead to genetic changes.

In May 2011, the U.S. Food and Drug Administration ordered the makers of all-metal replacements to study how frequently they fail, after Johnson & Johnson recalled one of the most problematic devices, the articular surface replacement. Then in February 2012 the *BMJ* reported that tens of thousands of patients with faulty replacements could have lasting, debilitating damage. "This is one very large, uncontrolled experiment exposing millions of patients to an unknown risk. We will only find out about the safety of these devices after large numbers of people have already been exposed," said Michael Carome, deputy director of Public Citizen's Health Research Group, in a release issued with the *BMJ* study's findings.

Your hip joints, just like the rest of your body, are self-repairing living organisms. When properly maintained, they will last a lifetime—replacement not required. Regular workouts—walking, dancing, biking, or swimming for twenty minutes a day—are a good way to exercise all the muscles of the hips and legs that support and help stabilize the hip joints. A diet of whole, unprocessed foods, and supplements such as glucosamine and chondroitin help prevent arthritis that can damage the hip joint. Likewise, good nutrition can help repair the joint. When faced with hip replacement surgery, consider other options. One is to help your body rebuild the joint. Other options include injections of hyaluronic acid, found naturally in joint fluid, to treat joint pain, and hip arthroscopy, a minimally invasive surgery to clean out the hip joint by trimming or removing loose cartilage or bone to reduce pain and the need for replacement. If you already have a metal implant, keep the stress off your hips by keeping your weight down, and do everything you can to boost your immune system to fight any impact from leaching metals.

Unfortunately, a lot of the abuse in the surgical profession is due to the overwhelming influence of the implant manufacturers. The doctors go along with it because it is profitable for them. If you are a surgeon, you don't earn a living by not doing surgery.

Antiaging Medicine Accelerates Aging

Conventional medicine treats aging as it does all disease—with mechanistic solutions, substituting surgery, drugs, and devices for the body's own repair systems. Not only does this approach not facilitate repairs, it destroys the cells' ability to repair and rejuvenate themselves. Older Americans are spending billions of dollars on hormone replacement therapies, elective surgery, and prescription lenses. What they are buying is cellular malfunction, accelerated aging, and more disease.

Aging, as commonly experienced, is really a disease that should be called *premature aging*, produced by accumulated repair deficits. Whether it shows up as wrinkled skin, failing eyesight, or a chronic disease, we age systemically, and fixing one outward sign of aging or another will never prevent or reverse aging. The root causes of our premature aging are deficiency and toxicity, the best way to stay biologically young is to address both of these by using the resources described in this book.

HRTs Crash Your Endocrine System

Hormone replacement therapy (HRT) is another medical mistake. Numerous studies have proven that HRT causes heart attack, stroke, and blood clots. Women on HRT are up to three times more likely to develop blood clots. After decades of well-founded suspicion, it has now been established that HRT causes cancer. A study of 46,000 women in a January 2000 issue of the *Journal of the American Medical Association* found that women who used the most common form of HRT for five years had a 40 percent increased risk of breast cancer. The risk increased by 8 percent with each year of use. A more recent study in the *Journal of the American Medical Association* (2010) found that not only does HRT increase the risk of breast cancer, but it makes it more likely that the cancer will be aggressive and deadly. A 2006 study in the *Journal of the National Cancer Institute* found a link between HRT and ovarian cancer; other studies have found links to lung cancer. Since 2000, many physicians have stopped prescribing HRT, and studies show that the recent decline in breast cancer deaths is the direct result. The breast cancer death rate is dropping because fewer doctors are giving their patients cancer!

Conventional Dentistry Fills You with Toxins

Conventional dentistry uses x-rays, toxic metals such as nickel and mercury, and carcinogenic local anesthetics. It is widely acknowledged that there is no safe level of radiation, yet dentists use x-rays routinely. Another routine dental procedure, the root canal, allows dangerous disease-causing bacteria to breed in your mouth. Even dental cleanings aren't generally safe or beneficial.

Cleanings

Dental cleanings remove plaque—a biological film that forms naturally over the surface of our teeth. Plaque is a complicated mixture of many kinds of bacteria, protein strands, other substances, fluids, and cells. Healthy alkaline plaque is essential for maintaining clean strong teeth. Its complex character gives plaque an extraordinary resistance to temperatures and corrosive liquids in the food. Healthy plaque fights intruding bacteria, provides essential ingredients for the enamel to heal itself, and also protects vital cells from temperature and chemical changes that occur during eating and drinking.

Today, in almost every dental office across the United States, a patient has a dental cleaning at each recall visit, at least twice a year. These treatments are prescribed without any evaluation as to whether they are necessary. If you have a buildup of hardened plaque around the edges of your teeth, removing these deposits reduces gum irritation. However, too much polishing of the teeth damages the delicate protective plaque layer on the tooth surface. In this way, a cleaning may cause teeth to become more porous and consequently more open to damage and decay.

Fillings

A so-called silver filling is actually about 50 percent mercury, one of the most dangerous toxins in our environment. Mercury damages the brain, central nervous system, immune system, and kidneys as well as causing cancer. Yet an estimated 100 million mercury fillings are still done annually in the United States. No one has ever been able to prove that there is a safe level of mercury. The EPA recommends ingesting a maximum of no more than 6.8 micrograms of mercury per day for a 150-pound person. Average daily absorption from fish and seafood is estimated at 2.3 micrograms. Alarmingly, a single mercury filling, through evaporation and mechanical wear, can release 15 micrograms per day, every day. A person with eight fillings will be absorbing 120 micrograms per day! Fortunately, plastic composites are now used extensively in place of mercury fillings. Anyone with mercury fillings should have them removed by a dentist who is skilled in the proper procedures for safe removal. You should have your own air supply during the removal so as not to breathe the mercury vapors.

Crowns

About 75 percent of porcelain crowns are made with a stainless-steel liner to give them strength. The stainless contains nickel. Nickel is an allergen and an even more powerful carcinogen than mercury. If you have porcelain crowns made with nickel, it would be best to remove them. Crowns made with gold are a better choice. Porcelain technology today has advanced to where crowns are available that have no metal at all; these would be the best choice.

Root Canals

Even though scientists have been warning us of the dangers of root canals for more than a century, conventional dentistry considers them safe. Yet virtually every root canal tooth has been found to be chronically infected. These low-grade infections produce toxins that poison the entire body, damaging immunity. Root-canalled teeth are essentially "dead" teeth that can become silent incubators for highly toxic anaerobic bacteria that, under certain conditions, make their way into your bloodstream and cause a number of diseases—some surfacing decades after the procedure. Most of these toxic teeth feel and look fine for many years, which makes their role in systemic disease even harder to trace. As long as your immune system remains strong, any bacteria that stray away from the infected tooth are captured and destroyed. But once your immune system is weakened by something like an accident, illness, or other trauma, your immune system may be unable to keep the infection in check. Then bacteria can migrate into the bloodstream and infect any organ, gland, or tissue.

The American Dental Association claims that root canals have been proven safe, but they have no published data or actual research to substantiate this claim. In fact, evidence is mounting to the contrary. Nearly every chronic degenerative disease has been linked with root canals, including heart disease; kidney disease; arthritis, joint, and rheumatic diseases; and autoimmune and neurological diseases, including lupus, ALS, and multiple sclerosis. Dr. George Meinig's 1993 book, *Root Canal Cover-Up*, continues to be the most comprehensive reference on this topic today.

Anesthetics

Local anesthetics (including lidocaine) are commonly used by dentists and may contribute substantially to our cancer epidemic. These anesthetics break down in the body into cancer-causing compounds called *anilines*. In 1993 the FDA found that lidocaine, when exposed to human tissue, breaks down into 2,6-dimethylaniline, an aniline that is known to cause virtually every kind of cancer in animals more than 99 percent of the time. In September 1996, because of these findings, the FDA removed from the market all over-the-counter painkillers containing local anesthetics and required that a warning be placed on all new prescription pharmaceuticals containing them. But existing prescription anesthetics were not required to carry the FDA's warning, so most health professionals are still unaware of this problem. To learn more, see Integrated Laboratory Systems' October 2000 report, *Final Toxicological Summary for Amide Local Anesthetics.* Fortunately, there is an anesthetic, Septocaine, that is not cancer causing, and you can request that your dentist use it.

Conclusion

Henry Bieler, M.D., author of *Food Is Your Best Medicine,* had good reason to say, "This is the dark age of medicine." Conventional allopathic medicine is less than 100 years old, but this fatally flawed system is a major cause of disease and has become our leading cause of death. It has failed to keep up with and put into practice the enormous advances in science over the last century, and has become corrupted by multinational drug and food industry interests that put their profits far ahead of improving your health and the human condition in general. It treats symptoms of disease and not causes. Its costs are horrendous because it doesn't cure anybody. Patients stay sick, and enormous sums of money are spent to keep treating them by suppressing their symptoms.

To avoid getting caught up in this flawed and dangerous system, keep your immunity strong with a good diet and high-quality supplements, and avoid toxins, including prescription drugs, vaccinations, and antibiotics. *The way to cure any disease is to address the problems of deficiency and toxicity and restore malfunctioning cells to normal.*

YOUR MAINTENANCE LIST
FOR THE MEDICAL PATHWAY:

Energy Production

Drugs—including antidepressants, anticonvulsants, anxiety meds, cholesterol meds, antibiotics, antiarrhythmics, antivirals, and cancer meds—are all toxic to mitochondria and inhibit energy production.

Inflammation

Do not take cholesterol-lowering statins. Inflammation is the cause of heart disease.

An anti-inflammatory diet, antioxidants, and omega-3 fats are more effective than statins.

Avoid vaccinations and other sources of aluminum, which accelerates inflammation.

Avoid elective surgery. It causes a substantial increase in inflammation.

Acid/Alkaline Balance

Most prescription drugs have an acidic effect on the body.

Digestive Health

Avoid antibiotics. They wipe out both good and bad intestinal flora.

Avoid anti-inflammatories and steroids. They harm the digestive tract.

Avoid colonoscopies. The preparation disrupts the intestinal flora.

Avoid birth control pills. They disrupt the normal balance of gut bacteria.

Take probiotics to restore the balance of good bacteria in the gut.

Hormonal Balance

Avoid hormone replacement therapy, which can cause heart attack, stroke, and cancer.

Avoid birth control pills; they seriously disrupt hormonal balance and cause disease.

Platelet Stickiness

Do not take aspirin to prevent blood clots; diet and supplements are safer and more effective.

Fat Storage

Drugs—especially birth control, antidepressant, and diabetes drugs—upset fat storage control and cause weight gain.

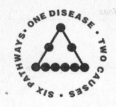

TWELVE

The Bottom Line

The doctor of the future will give no medicine,
but will interest his patients in the care of the human frame,
in diet, and in the cause and prevention of disease.

—Thomas Edison

Each person carries his own doctor inside him.
They come to us not knowing that truth.
We are at our best when we give the doctor who resides
in each patient a chance to go to work.

—Albert Schweitzer

Things that we value most like family, health,
freedom, wealth, and happiness—do not exist without
sustainability. In other words, if we don't learn how
to live sustainably, life will soon be nothing more than
a hell on Earth for those few of us who survive.

—J. Morris Hicks

We are in the midst of a healthcare crisis, going broke trying to pay for the costs of health care. This crisis is the result of the combined effects of an aging population, an epidemic of chronic disease, and steeply rising treatment costs. More than 10,000 baby boomers are retiring *every day*, putting unprecedented stress on the U.S. federal budget. To pay for these costs, our government is printing and borrowing money hand over fist. Our young will be taxed unmercifully to pay back what we are borrowing; they are in danger of becoming the first generation in our history to have a lower standard of living than their parents. With all of the industrialized countries going bankrupt trying to pay for the cost of disease, the threat of a catastrophic economic collapse is imminent. Denying care, lowering payments to doctors, and printing money are not viable long-term solutions.

The win-win solution is to cut costs by ending the epidemic of chronic disease, the so-called diseases of aging such as Alzheimer's, arthritis, cancer, diabetes, heart disease, and osteoporosis. We already know how to end this epidemic. All we have to do is educate ourselves and put this knowledge to use.

However, there are obstacles to be overcome—powerful interests that will do everything they can to stand in the way. Drug companies and the entire disease industry prosper only when millions of people get sick and stay sick. Allied against progress are the food, chemical, agriculture, GMO, personal care product, home furnishing, telecommunication, and other industries that are in no rush to make the substantial changes needed to support society's health.

Such interests reinforce a medical education system stuck in a seventeenth-century view of the body as a machine and in the notion that symptoms of ill health need to be treated with expensive drugs and surgery. The self-healing capacity of the body is ignored, along with the effects of our diet, mind, spirit, emotions, environment, and lifestyle.

The radical change needed will not come from the top down. It will have to come from the bottom up, starting with *you*. By paying attention to your maintenance items and moving yourself toward health on each of the Six Pathways, you can choose health for yourself. Then, by telling others of your success, you can help to start a revolution that can end the healthcare crisis.

How to maintain good health is not a mystery. *The human body is a self-regulating, self-repairing system.* A healthy lifestyle is the most powerful medicine in the universe. Thousands of studies have shown that if you eat a good diet, get regular exercise, maintain a healthy weight, reduce your stress, and don't smoke or take drugs, you will reduce your risk of developing a chronic disease by *at least* 80 percent! Imagine the economic impact of reducing healthcare costs by 80 percent. Yet how many people follow such a healthy lifestyle? *The estimates are less than 4 percent.*

Few people today know that health is a choice, and even fewer know how to make that choice. We have been trained to believe that we don't have to do anything special to maintain health, and that if we do get sick, we can go to a doctor who will give us a magic pill and make our problems go away. We even expect society to foot the bill for these services. We need to start holding each other accountable for making poor choices that result in preventable illness.

But people can't make responsible choices if they don't know how. Most people are overwhelmed and confused by the constant flood of conflicting health information and the thousands of different diseases that physicians "treat" with drugs and surgery. They end up feeling powerless because they have no idea why they got sick or how to make themselves well again.

However, my approach cuts through the confusion by focusing on the ultimate causes of disease. By preventing and reversing disease through the Six Pathways, you put into your own hands the power to get healthy and stay healthy. This approach is based on solid science and the experience of thousands who have already benefitted from learning and implementing the Beyond Health model.

If I had this level of understanding when I was younger, I would never have experienced the illness that came close to taking my life thirty years ago. Only by using my scientific background to acquire this understanding was I able to save my life and restore my health. My fervent wish is that what I have learned and shared with you in this book will help you to do the same.

All you need to know at any point in time is which direction you are going along each of the pathways—toward health or disease—and to make corrections. You cannot make good choices along only one or two of the pathways and expect to achieve optimal health; this approach limits many health plans and books, useful though they may be. Many approaches are on the right track, but they do not look at the whole picture. Making healthy choices with respect to all of the Six Pathways is what empowers the body to do the maintenance it needs to self-regulate, repair, and balance itself.

That said, each choice you make in a positive direction, toward health, on any Pathway, at any time, will improve your life. Each step toward health puts you closer to your true potential and further away from the risk of disease or illness. Each contribution, no matter how small, is significant. Don't be intimidated by all the changes you need to make; make the changes you can and keep improving over time. The important thing is that you start doing *something*.

Today, most of us are doing most things wrong most of the time, and it is making us sick and killing us. Turn that around. Start doing most things right most of the time, and it will be like a miracle. You don't have to be a fanatic, and you don't have to be perfect. Just make the right choices most of the time instead of the wrong ones. It's never too late to start. An old car can be restored with some tender loving care, and so can you. Almost anyone can become healthier and biologically younger by doing the proper maintenance.

While individual responsibility alone is sufficient to cut healthcare costs significantly, government action would also be helpful and is needed. Unfortunately, the government does much to cause and perpetuate disease. For example, we know that sugar is a deadly metabolic poison and a major cause of disease, yet the federal government subsidizes the sugar industry with price controls. Instead, sugar should be outlawed like cocaine or, at the very least, be regulated like alcohol and tobacco. Children are not allowed to purchase alcohol and tobacco, yet they are allowed to purchase products containing sugar, which is far more dangerous and damaging to their health. Milk is not a healthy food, yet the government subsidizes the dairy industry. Fluoride is a deadly metabolic poison, yet governments mandate that it be added to the water supply. Glutamates are allowed in foods, but they should be outlawed. Vaccinations damage health but are mandated by government. The government allows dentists to put deadly mercury in your mouth. Microwave ovens are allowed to be sold without proper warnings about their danger to health. Cell phone towers are allowed to be placed near schools, dwellings, and businesses, disregarding the research showing how such installations damage health. The FDA is an out-of-control government agency that contributes to disease by protecting the drug industry, which causes and perpetuates disease, while persecuting the vitamin industry, which prevents and cures disease. The government can reduce the cost of disease by simply not causing so much of it.

Government also needs to get out of the way and allow innovation in medicine. Certain procedures are written into the law. For example, in California, the only legal treatments for cancer are treatments that don't work: chemotherapy, surgery, and radiation. It is a felony for a doctor to use other treatments, despite abundant scientific evidence that they are safe and more effective. This is why the cancer death rate is the same today as it was in 1950. No progress has been made. Progress is impossible when ineffective treatments are written into the law.

Health is a choice not yet chosen. Yet to save ourselves and our economy, we must give health a chance. Embark on a journey of learning and understanding that can empower you to get well and stay well. Choose health for yourself, become an example to others, and help to create the massive social change we need. . . .

Here's to your *choice*!

APPENDIX A

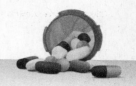

About Beyond Health International

Beyond Health International is an internationally respected source of health education, supplements, and health products of exceptional quality—one of a handful of high-end suppliers. Beyond Health's mission is to help you to go *beyond health* as you have known it, and its passionate commitment to quality puts it in a class of its own. Beyond Health's formulations provide more biologically correct and active nutrients per dollar than lower-priced products, and therefore deliver the lowest cost and highest possible value to its customers. The most expensive vitamin you can buy is one that doesn't work because it's not made with biologically correct ingredients. With supplements, high quality means high purity and high biological activity, supplying your body with what it needs to get well and stay well. High-quality ingredients cost more, but they are so much more biologically active, they deliver the most nutrients to your cells at the least cost.

In addition to health information, vitamins, minerals, and other supplements, Beyond Health also supplies high-quality food products such as coconut oil and olive oil. It also provides reverse-osmosis water filters, whole-house water filters, and Beyond Health–approved personal care products, rebounders, and saunas.

Call one of our wellness consultants for assistance with your needs. Contact Beyond Health at:

www.beyondhealth.com • *info@beyondhealth.com*
800-250-3063 (United States and Canada only) • 954-492-1324

APPENDIX B

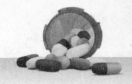

Foods with Acidic Effect
on Body Chemistry

Food Category	Lowest Acid	Low Acid	More Acid	Most Acid
Spices/Herbs	Curry	Vanilla	Nutmeg	Pudding/Jam/Jelly
Preservatives	*MSG*	Benzoate	Aspartame	*Table Salt (NaCl)*
Beverages	*Kona Coffee*	Alcohol Black Tea	*Coffee*	Beer Soda Yeast/Hops/Malt
Sweeteners	Honey Maple Syrup		*Saccharin*	Sugar Cocoa
Vinegar	Rice Vinegar	Balsamic Vinegar	Red Wine Vinegar	White/Acetic Vinegar
Therapeutic		*Antihistamines*	*Psychotropics*	*Antibiotics*
Processed Dairy	Cream/Butter Yogurt Goat Cheese Sheep Cheese	Cow Milk Aged Cheese Soy Cheese Goat Milk	• Casein/Milk Protein Cottage Cheese New Cheese Soy Milk	*Processed Cheese* Ice Cream
Eggs	Chicken Egg			
Meat and Game	Gelatin Organs • Venison	Lamb/Mutton • Boar • Elk	Pork Veal • Bear	Beef
Fish and Shellfish	Fish	Shellfish Mollusks	• Mussel • Squid	• Lobster
Fowl	Wild Duck	Goose Turkey	Chicken	Pheasant
Grains, Cereals, and Grasses	• Triticale Millet Kasha • Amaranth Brown Rice	Buckwheat Wheat • Spelt/Teff/Kamut Farina/Semolina White Rice	Maize Barley Goat Corn Rye Oat Bran	Barley Processed Flour

• Therapeutic, gourmet, or exotic items   Italicized items are NOT recommended foods

Foods wih Acidic Effect on Body Chemistry (continued)

Food Category	Lowest Acid	Low Acid	More Acid	Most Acid
Nuts, Seeds, Sprouts, and Oils	Pine Nut Pumpkin Seed Oil Sunflower Seed Oil Canola Oil	Almond Oil Seasame Oil Safflower Oil Tapioca • Seitan or Tofu	Pecan Pistachio Seed Chestnut Oil Lard Palm Kernel Oil	Hazelnut Walnut Brazil Nut •*Cottonseed Oil/* *Meal*
Beans and Vegetables	Fava Bean Kidney Bean Black-eyed Pea Spinach String/Wax Bean Zucchini Chutney Rhubarb	Split Pea Pinto Bean White Bean Navy/Red Bean Aduki Bean Lima or Mung Bean Chard	Green Pea Peanut Snow Peas Legumes (other) Chick Pea Garbanzo Carrot	Soybean Carob
Fruit	Coconut Guava • Pickled Fruit Dried Fruit Fig Persimmon Juice • Cherimoya Date	Plum Prune Tomato	Cranberry Pomegranate	

• Therapeutic, gourmet, or exotic items   Italicized items are NOT recommended Foods

Foods with Alkaline Effect
on Body Chemistry

Food Category	Most Alkaline	More Alkalin	Low Alkaline	Lowest Alkaline
Spices/Herbs	Baking Soda	Spices Cinnamon Licorice • Black Cohash Agave	• Herbs (most): Arnica Bergamot Echinacea Chrysanthemum Ephedra Feverfew Goldenseal Lemongrass Aloe Vera Nettle Angelica	White Willow Bark Slippery Elm Artemisia Annual
Preservatives	*Sea Salt*			*Sulfite*
Beverages **Sweeteners** **Vinegar** **Therapeutic** **Processed Dairy**	Mineral Water • Umebosh Plum	• Kambucha *Molasses* Soy Sauce	• Green or Mu Tea Rice Syrup Apple Cider Vinegar Sake	Ginger Tea Sucanat • Umeboshi Vinegar Algae, Blue Green Ghee (Clarified Butter) Human Breast Milk
Eggs **Meat and Game** **Fish/Shellfish**			• Quail Egg	• Duck Egg
Fowl				

• Therapeutic, gourmet, or exotic items

Foods with Alkaline Effect on Body Chemistry (continued)

Food Category	Most Alkaline	More Alkaline	Low Alkaline	Lowest Alkaline
Beans and Vegetables	Lentil Brocoflower • Seaweed Noral/Kombu/ Wakame / Hijiki Onion / Miso • Daikon / Taro Root • Sea Vegetables (other) Dandelion Green • Burdock • Lotus Root Sweet Potato/Yam	Kohlrabi Parsnip/Taro Garlic Asparagus Kale Parsley Endive Arugula Mustard Greens Jerusalem Artichoke Ginger Root Broccoli	Potato Bell Pepper Mushroom Fungi Cauliflower Cabbage Rutabaga • Salsify/Ginseng Eggplant Pumpkin Collard Greens	Brussels Sprout Beet Chive Cilantro Celery Scallion Okra Cucumber Turnip Greens Squash Artichoke Lettuce Jicama
Fruits	Lime Nectarine Persimmon Raspberry Watermelon Tangerine Pineapple	Grapefruit Cantaloupe Honeydew Citrus Olive • Dewberry Loganberry Mango	Lemon Pear Avocado Apple Blackberry Cherry Peach Papaya	Orange Apricot Banana Blueberry Pineapple Juice • Raisin/Currant Grape Strawberry

• Therapeutic, gourmet, or exotic items

BIBLIOGRAPHY

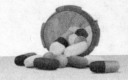

Adams, K.M., et al. "Nutrition education in U.S. medical schools: Latest update of a national survey." *Academic Medicine* (2010) 85 (9): 1537–1542.

Advisory Committee on Immunization Practices. "Updated recommendations for use of Tetanus toxoid, reduced diphtheria toxoid and acellular pertussis (Tdap) vaccine." *Centers for Disease Control and Prevention, Morbidity and Mortality Weekly* (2011) 60 (01): 13–15.

Age-Related Eye Disease Study Research Group. "A randomized, placebo-controlled, clinical trial of high-dose supplementation with vitamins C and E, beta carotene, and zinc for age-related macular degeneration and vision loss: AREDS report no. 8." *Archives of Ophthalmology* (2001) 119 (10): 1417–1436.

Alavania, M.C., et al. "Increased cancer burden among pesticide applicators and others due to pesticide exposure." *CA: A Cancer Journal for Clinicians* (2013) 63 (2): 120–142.

Alford, L. "What men should know about the impact of physical activity on their health." *International Journal of Clinical Practice* (2010) 64 (13): 1731.

Allen, M. "Assembly-line colonoscopies at clinic described." *Las Vegas Sun*, March 9, 2008; accessed January 29, 2013, http://www.lasvegassun.com/news/2008/mar/09/assembly-line-colonoscopies-clinic-described/.

American Cancer Society. "American Cancer Society guidelines for the early detection of cancer" accessed January 29, 2013, http://www.cancer.org/healthy/findcancerearly/cancerscreeningguidelines/american-cancer-society-guidelines-for-the-early-detection-of-cancer.

Ames, B. "Micronutrient deficiencies: A major cause of DNA damage." *Annals of the New York Academy of Sciences* (1999) 889 (1): 87–106.

———. "Micronutrients prevent cancer and delay aging." Paper presented at the Strang International Cancer Prevention Conference, New York City, 1998.

Anderson, R. "Toxic emissions from carpets." *Journal of Nutritional and Environmental Medicine* (1995) 5: 375–386.

Andrew, B., et al. "Meditation effects on cognitive function and cerebral blood flow in subjects with memory loss: A preliminary study." *Journal of Alzheimer's Disease* (2010) 20 (2): 517–526.

Angell, M. *The truth about the drug companies: How they deceive us and what to do about it.* New York: Random House, 2005.

Appleton, N. *Lick the sugar habit.* Garden City Park, NY: Avery Publishing Group, 1996.

Arhant-Sudhir, K., et al. "Pet ownership and cardiovascular risk reduction: Supporting evidence, conflicting data, and underlying mechanisms." *Clinical and Experimental Pharmacology and Physiology* (2011) 38 (11): 734–738.

Aris, A., and Leblanc, S. "Maternal and fetal exposure to pesticides associated to genetically modified foods in Eastern Townships of Quebec, Canada." *Reproductive Toxicology* (2011) 31 (4): 528–533.

Armanios, M., et al. "Short telomeres are sufficient to cause the degenerative defects associated with aging." *American Journal of Human Genetics* (2009) 85 (6): 823–832.

Armstrong, B., and Doll, R. "Environmental factors and cancer incidence and mortality in different countries, with special reference to dietary practices." *International Journal of Cancer* (1975) 15 (4): 617–631.

Arnetz, B.B., et al. "The effects of 884 MHz GSM wireless communication signals on self-reported symptom and sleep (EEG)—An experimental provocation study." *PIERS Online* (2007) 3 (7): 1148–1150.

Auso, E., et al. "A moderate and transient deficiency of maternal thyroid function at the beginning of fetal neocorticogenesis alters neuronal migration." *Endocrinology* (2004) 145 (9): 4037–4047.

Baillie-Hamilton, P. *Toxic overload.* New York: Avery, Penguin, 2005.

Balfour, E. *The living soil.* New York: Universe Books, 1976.

Barbagallo, M., et al. "Magnesium homeostasis and aging." *Magnesium Research* (2009) 22 (4): 235–246.

Barclay, R.L., et al. "Colonoscopic withdrawal times and adenoma detection during screening colonoscopy." *New England Journal of Medicine* (2006) 355 (24): 2533–2541.

Beasley, J.D., and Swift, J.J. *The Kellogg report*. Annandale-on-Hudson, NY: Institute of Health Policy and Practice, Bard College Center, 1989.

Bebeshko, V., et al. "Does ionizing radiation accelerate the aging phenomena?" *Twenty Years after Chernobyl Accident: Future Outlook*. Conference paper, Kiev, Ukraine, April 24–26, 2006. Contributed Papers (HOLTEH, Kiev) 1:13–18.

Becker, R.O., and Selden, G. *The body electric: Electromagnetism and the foundation of life*. New York: William Morrow, 1985.

Beecher, H.K. "The powerful placebo." *Journal of the American Medical Association* (1955) 159 (17): 1602–1606.

Beetz, A., et al. "Psychosocial and psychophysiological effects of human-animal interactions: The possible role of oxytocin." *Frontiers in Psychology* (2012) 3: 234.

Berkrot, B., and Pierson, R. "FDA adds diabetes, memory loss warnings to statins." Reuters, February 28, 2012; accessed January 29, 2013, http://www.reuters.com/article/2012/02/28/us-fda-statins-idUSTRE81R1O220120228.

Bernstein, I.L., et al. "Immune responses in farm workers after exposure to Bacillus thuringiensis pesticides." *Environmental Health Perspectives* (1999) 107 (7): 575–582.

Bibbins-Domingo, K., et al. "Projected effect of dietary salt reductions on future cardiovascular disease." *New England Journal of Medicine* (2010) 362 (7): 590–599.

Bieler, H. *Food is your best medicine*. New York: Ballantine Books, 1987.

Blair, S.N., and Church, T.S. "The fitness, obesity, and health equation: Is physical activity the common denominator?" *Journal of the American Medical Association* (2004) 292 (10): 1232–1234.

Blaylock, R.L. *Excitotoxins*. Santa Fe: Health Press, 1997.

———. *Health and nutrition secrets that can save your life*. Albuquerque: Health Press, 2002.

———. *Natural strategies for cancer patients*. New York: Kensington, 2003.

Bloom, M., et al. "Environmental exposure to PBDEs and thyroid function among New York anglers." *Environmental Toxicology and Pharmacology* (2007) 25 (3): 386–392.

Bocio, A., et al. "Polybrominated diphenyl ethers (DBDEs) in foodstuffs: Human exposure through diet." *Journal of Agricultural Food Chemistry* (2003) 51 (10): 3191–3195.

Bone, E., et al. "The production of urinary phenols by gut bacteria and their possible role in the causation of large bowel cancer." *American Journal of Clinical Nutrition* (1976) 29 (12): 1448–1454.

Boutwell, R.K., and Bosch, D.K. "The tumor-promoting action of phenol and related compounds for mouse skin." *Cancer Research* (1959) 19: 413–424.

Bowman, G.L., et al. "Nutrient biomarker patterns, cognitive function, and MRI measures of brain aging." *Neurology* (2012) 78 (4): 241–249.

Boyle, C.A., et al. "Trends in the prevalence of developmental disabilities in US children, 1997–2008." *Pediatrics* (2011) 127 (6): 1034–1042.

Braune, S., et al. "Resting blood pressure increase during exposure to a radio-frequency electromagnetic field." *Lancet* (1998) 351 (9119): 1857–1858.

Bravo, J.A., et al. "Ingestion of Lactobacillus strain regulates emotional behavior and central GABA receptor expression in a mouse via the vagus nerve." *Proceedings of the National Academy of Sciences* (2011) 108 (38): 16050–16055.

Brekhman, I.I., and Nesterenko, I.F. *Brown sugar and health*. New York: Pergamon Press, 1983.

Brenner, D.J., and Elliston, C.D. "Estimated radiation risks potentially associated with full-body CT screening." *Radiology* (2004) 232 (3): 735–738.

Brinton, L.A., et al. "Oral contraceptives and breast cancer risk among younger women." *Journal of the National Cancer Institute* (1995) 87 (13): 827–835.

Brouilette, S.W., et al. "Telomere length, risk of coronary heart disease, and statin treatment in the West of Scotland Primary Prevention Study: A nested case-control study." *Lancet* (2007) 369 (9556): 81–82.

Burton, G.W., et al. "Human plasma and tissue alpha-tocopherol concentrations in response to supplementation with deuterated natural and synthetic vitamin E." *American Journal of Clinical Nutrition* (1998) 67 (4): 669–684.

Buxton, J.L., et al. "Childhood obesity is associated with shorter leukocyte telomere length." *Journal of Clinical Endocrinology and Metabolism* (2011) 96 (5): 1500–1505.

Canela, A., et al. "High-throughput telomere length quantification by FISH and its application to human population studies." *Proceedings of the National Academy of Sciences* (2007) 104 (13): 5300–5305.

Casdorph, R., and Walker, M. *Toxic metal syndrome*. Garden City Park, NY: Avery Publishing Group, 1995.

Cawthon, R.M., et al. "Association between telomere length in blood and mortality in people aged 60 years or older." *Lancet* (2003) 361 (9355): 393–395.

Centers for Disease Control. *Childhood obesity facts*. Accessed March 12, 2013, http://www.cdc.gov/healthy youth/obesity/facts.htm.

———. *Fourth national report on human exposure to environmental chemicals*. Atlanta, GA: U.S. Department of Health and Human Services, 2009, http://www.cdc.gov/exposurereport/.

Chan, J.M., et al. "Dairy products, calcium, and prostate cancer risk in the Physicians' Health Study." *American Journal of Clinical Nutrition* (2001) 74 (4): 549–554.

Chaufan, G., et al. "Glyphosate commercial formulation causes cytotoxicity, oxidative effects, and apoptosis on human cells: Differences with its active ingredient." *International Journal of Toxicology* (2014) 33 (1): 29–38.

Chen, C.L., et al. "Hormone replacement therapy in relation to breast cancer." *Journal of the American Medical Association* (2002) 287 (6): 734–741.

Cheraskin, E., et al. *The vitamin C connection*. New York: Bantam Books, 1983.

Cherkas, L., et al. "The association between physical activity in leisure time and leukocyte telomere length." *Archives of Internal Medicine* (2008) 168 (2): 154–158.

Chevrier, J., et al. "Polybrominated diphenyl ether (PBDE) flame retardants and thyroid hormone during pregnancy." *Environmental Health Perspectives* (2010) 118 (10): 1444–1449.

———. "Associations between prenatal exposure to polychlorinated biphenyls and neonatal thyroid-stimulating hormone levels in a Mexican-American population, Salinas Valley, California." *Environmental Health Perspectives* (2007) 115 (10): 1490–1496.

Chien, L.C., et al. "Hair mercury concentration and fish consumption: Risk and perception of risk among women of childbearing age." *Environmental Research* (2010) 110 (1): 123–129.

Chlebowski, R.T., et al. "Estrogen plus progestin and breast cancer incidence and mortality in postmenopausal women." *Journal of the American Medical Association* (2010) 304 (15): 1684–1692.

Chopra, D. *Ageless body, timeless mind*. New York: Harmony Books, 1993.

———. *Creating Health*. Boston: Houghton Mifflin, 1987.

———. *Quantum Healing*. New York: Bantam Books, 1989.

Clarke, J.D. *Prostate cancer prevention with broccoli: From cellular to human studies*. Ann Arbor: ProQuest, UMI Dissertation Publishing, 2012.

Clinton, S.K., et al. "Effects of ammonium acetate and sodium cholate on N-methyl-N'-nitro-N-nitrosoguanidine-induced colon carcinogenesis of rats." *Cancer Research* (1988) 48 (11): 3035–3039.

Cohen, A.M., et al. "Change of diet of Yemenite Jews in relation to diabetes and ischaemic heart-disease." *Lancet* (1961) 2 (7217): 1399–1401.

Cohen, R. *Milk: The deadly poison*. Englewood Cliffs, NJ: Argus, 1997.

Colagar, A.H. "Zinc levels in seminal plasma are associated with sperm quality in fertile and infertile men." *Nutritional Research* (2009) 29 (2): 82–88.

Colbert, D. *Toxic relief: Restore health and energy through fasting and detoxification*. Lake Mary, FL: Siloam, 2003.

Committee on Quality of Health Care in America and Institute of Medicine. *Crossing the quality chasm: A new health system for the 21st Century*. Washington, D.C.: National Academies Press, 2001.

Comstock, G.W., and Partridge, K.B. "Church attendance and health." *Journal of Chronic Disease* (1972) 25 (12): 665–672.

Congcong, H., et al. "Exercise-induced BCL2-regulated autophagy is required for muscle glucose homeostasis." *Nature* (2012) 481 (7382): 511–515.

"Consultatus Interruptus." *Internal Medicine News and Cardiology News* (1993) December: 9.

Corpet, D.E., et al. "Colonic protein fermentation and promotion of colon carcinogenesis by thermolyzed casein." *Nutrition and Cancer* (1995) 23 (3): 271–281.

———. "Promotion of colonic microadenoma growth in mice and rats fed cooked sugar or cooked casein and fat." *Cancer Research* (1990) 50 (21): 6955–6958.

Costello, L.C., et al. "Decreased zinc and downregulation of ZIP3 zinc uptake transporter in the development of pancreatic adenocarcinoma." *Cancer Biology and Therapy* (2011) 12 (4): 297–303.

Costenbader, K.H., et al. "Immunosenescence and rheumatoid arthritis: Does telomere shortening predict impending disease?" *Autoimmunity Reviews* (2011) 10 (9): 569–573.

Coulter, H. *Vaccination, social violence and criminality: The medical assault on the American brain.* Berkeley, CA: North Atlantic Books, 1990.

Cousins, N. *Anatomy of an illness.* New York: Bantam, 1979.

Cummins, R., and Lilliston, B. *Genetically engineered food.* New York: Marlow, 2000.

Dadd, D.L. *Nontoxic and natural.* Los Angeles: Jeremy P. Tarcher, 1984.

Dallaire, R., et al. "Thyroid function and plasma concentrations of polyhalogenated compounds in Inuit adults." *Environmental Health Perspectives* (2009) 117 (9): 1380–1386.

Das, R.R., and Singh, M. "Oral zinc for the common cold." *Journal of the American Medical Association* (2014) 311 (14): 1440–1441.

de Gonzalez, A.B., et al. "Projected cancer risks from computed tomographic scans performed in the United States in 2007." *Archives of Internal Medicine* (2009) 169 (22): 2071–2077.

Dean, C. *Death by modern medicine.* New York: Matrix Verite Media, 2005.

Deardorff, J. "What berries can do for you." *Chicago Tribune News*, March 2, 2011; accessed January 29, 2013, http://articles.chicagotribune.com/2011-03-02/health/sc-health-0302-berries-health-effects20110302_1_blueberries-bladder-infections-health-benefits.

Dei Cas, A., et al. "Lower endothelial progenitor cell number, family history of cardiovascular disease and reduced HDL-cholesterol levels are associated with shorter leukocyte telomere length in healthy young adults." *Nutrition, Metabolism, and Cardiovascular Diseases* (2013) 23 (3): 272–278.

Dethlefsen, L., and Relman, D.A. "Incomplete recovery and individualized responses of the human distal gut microbiota to repeated antibiotic perturbation." *Proceedings of the National Academy of Sciences* (2011) 108 (Suppl 1): 4554–4561.

Devore, E.E., et al. "Dietary intakes of berries and flavonoids in relation to cognitive decline." *Annals of Neurology* (2012) 72 (1): 135–143.

———. "Relative telomere length and cognitive decline in the Nurses' Health Study." *Neuroscience Letters* (2011) 492 (1): 15–18.

Diamond, H. *Fit for life: A new beginning.* New York: Kensington, 2000.

Diez, S., et al. "Prenatal and early childhood exposure to mercury and methylmercury in Spain, a high fish consumer country." *Archives of Environmental Contamination and Toxicology* (2009) 56 (3): 615–622.

Dolecek, T.A., and Grandits, G. "Dietary polyunsaturated fatty acids and mortality in the Multiple Risk Factor Intervention Trial (MRFIT)." *World Review of Nutrition and Dietetics* (1991) 66: 205–16.

Dossey, L. *The power of prayer and the practice of medicine.* San Francisco: Harper, 1993.

Du, M., et al. "Physical activity, sedentary behavior, and leukocyte telomere length in women." *American Journal of Epidemiology* (2012) 175 (5): 414–422.

Dufault, R., et al. "Mercury from chlor-alkali plants: Measured concentrations in food product sugar." *Environmental Health* (2009) 8 (1): 2.

Edwards, J. "Lawsuit claims Pfizer deceived doctors into prescribing its cholesterol drug Lipitor." CBSnews.com, February 11, 2010; accessed May 26, 2012, http://www.cbsnews.com/8301-505123_162-42844207/lawsuit-claims-pfizer-deceived-doctors-into-prescribing-its-cholesterol-drug-lipitor/.

Eger, H., et al. "The influence of being physically near to a cell phone transmission mast on the incidence of cancer." *Umwelt Medizin Gesellschaft* (2004) 17 (4): 326–332.

Ensminger, A., et al. *Food and nutrition encyclopedia.* Clovis, CA: Pegus Press, 1983.

Environmental Protection Agency, *Pesticide Industry Sales and Usage, 2006–2007 Market Estimates.*

Environmental Working Group. "Chromium-6 is widespread in US tap water," December 20, 2010; accessed January 29, 2013, http://www.ewg.org/chromium6-in-tap-water.

———. "Testing finds hundreds of contaminants in America's drinking water," December 2009; accessed January 29, 2013, http://www.ewg.org/tap-water/reportfindings.

Epel, E.S., et al. "Accelerated telomere shortening in response to life stress." *Proceedings of the National Academy of Sciences* (2004) 101 (49): 17312–17315.

Epstein, L.J., and Mardon, S. *The Harvard Medical School guide to a good night's sleep.* New York: McGraw Hill, 2006.

Erasmus, U. *Fats and Oils.* Vancouver: Alive Books, 1986.

———. *Fats that heal, fats that kill.* Bumaby, Canada: Alive Books, 1993.

Ershoff, B.H. "Synergistic toxicity of food additives in rats fed a diet low in dietary fiber." *Journal of Food Science* (1976) 41 (4): 949–951.

Escrich, E., et al. "Olive oil, an essential component of the Mediterranean Diet, and breast cancer." *Public Health Nutrition* (2011) 14 (12): 2323–2332.

Espel, E., et al. "The rate of leukocyte telomere shortening predicts mortality from cardiovascular disease in elderly men." *AGING* (2008) 1 (1): 81–88.

Fallon, S., with Enig, M.G. *Nourishing traditions: The cookbook that challenges politically correct nutrition and the diet dictocrats.* Washington, D.C.: New Trends, 2000.

Fälth-Magnusson, K., and Mangusson, K.E. "Elevated levels of serum antibodies to the lectin wheat germ agglutinin in celiac children lend support to the gluten-lectin theory of celiac disease." *Pediatric Allergy and Immunology* (1995) 6 (2): 98–102.

Farzaneh-Far, R., et al. "Association of marine omega-3 fatty acid levels with telomeric aging in patients with coronary heart disease." *Journal of the American Medical Association* (2010) 303 (3): 250–257.

Finamore, A., et al. "Intestinal and peripheral immune response to MON810 maize ingestion in weaning and old mice." *Journal of Agricultural and Food Chemistry* (2008) 56 (23): 11533–11539.

Fletcher, T., et al. "Associations between PFOA, PFOS, and changes in the expression of genes involved in cholesterol metabolism in humans." *Environment International* (2013) 57–58: 2–10.

Foster, H. "Lifestyle changes and the spontaneous regression of cancer: An initial computer analysis." *International Journal of Biosocial Research* (1988) 10 (1): 17–33.

Fowler, S., et al. "Diet soft drink consumption is associated with increased waist circumference in the San Antonio Longitudinal Study of Aging." Abstract presented at the annual meeting of the American Diabetes Association, San Diego, CA, June 24–28, 2011, Abstract No. 62-OR.

Francis, R. *Never be fat again.* Deerfield Beach, FL: Health Communications, 2007.

———. *Never be sick again.* Deerfield Beach, FL: Health Communications, 2002.

———. *Never fear cancer again.* Deerfield Beach, FL: Health Communications, 2011.

———. *Never feel old again.* Deerfield Beach, FL: Health Communications, 2013.

Friedman, H.S., et al. "Personality and health, subjective well-being, and longevity." *Journal of Personality* (2010) 78: 179–215.

Fujimura, K.E., et al. "House dust exposure mediates gut microbiome *Lactobacillus* enrichment and airway immune defense against allergens and virus infection." *Proceedings of the National Academy of Sciences Early Edition*, December 16, 2013, www.pnas.org/cgi/doi/10.1073/pnas.1310750111.

Gardener, H., et al. "Diet soft drink consumption is associated with an increased risk of vascular events in the Northern Manhattan Study." *Journal of General Internal Medicine* (2012) 27 (9): 1120–1126.

George, M.G., et al. "Trends in stroke hospitalizations and associated risk factors among children and young adults, 1995–2008." *Annals of Neurology* (2011) 70 (5): 713–721.

Godfrey, R.J., et al. "The exercise-induced growth hormone response in athletes." *Sports Medicine* (2003) 33 (8): 599–613.

Gofman, J.W. *Radiation from medical procedures in the pathogenesis of cancer and ischemic heart disease: Dose-response studies with physicians per 100,000 population.* San Francisco: Committee for Nuclear Responsibility, 1999.

Goldberg, B., et al. *Alternative medicine: The definitive guide.* Tiburon, CA: Future Medicine Publishing, 1993.

Goldner, W.S., et al. "Pesticide use and thyroid disease among women in the Agricultural Health Study." *American Journal of Epidemiology* (2010) 171 (4): 455–464.

Golomb, B. "Effects of statins on energy and fatigue with exertion: Results from a randomized controlled trial." *Archives of Internal Medicine* (2012) 172 (15): 1180–1182.

———. "Statin adverse effects: A review of the literature and evidence for a mitochondrial mechanism." *American Journal of Cardiovascular Drugs* (2008) 8 (6): 373–418.

Grandjean, P., et al. "Serum vaccine antibody concentrations in children exposed to perfluorinated compounds." *Journal of the American Medical Association* (2012) 307 (4): 391–397.

Green, D.R., et al. "Mitochondria and the autophagy-inflammation-cell death axis in organismal aging." *Science* (2011) 333 (6046): 1109–1112.

Gunderson, E.L. "FDA Total Diet Study, April 1982–April 1984, dietary intakes of pesticides, selected elements, and other chemicals." *Journal of the Association of Official Analytical Chemists* (1988) 71 (6): 1200–1209.

Guzyeyeva, G.V. "Lectin glycosylation as a marker of thin gut inflammation." *FASEB Journal* (2008) 22: 898.3.

Haddow, J.E., et al. "Maternal thyroid deficiency during pregnancy and subsequent neuropsychological development of the child." *New England Journal of Medicine* (1999) 341 (8): 549–555.

Haley, B.E. "Mercury toxicity: Genetic susceptibility and synergistic effects." *Medical Veritas* (2005) 2: 535–542.

Haley, D. *Politics in healing.* Washington, D.C.: Potomac Valley Press, 2000.

Halldorsson, T.I., et al. "Intake of artificially sweetened soft drinks and risk of preterm delivery: A prospective cohort study in 59,334 Danish pregnant women." *American Journal of Clinical Nutrition* (2010) 92 (3): 626–633.

Harbige, L. "Fatty acids, the immune response, and autoimmunity: A question of n-6 essentiality and the balance between n-6 and n-3." *Lipids* (2003) 38 (4): 323–341.

Harley, C.B., et al. "A natural product telomerase activator as part of a health maintenance program." *Rejuvenation Research* (2011) 14 (1): 45–56.

Harley, K.G., et al. "PBDE concentrations in women's serum and fecundability." *Environmental Health Perspectives* (2010) 118 (5): 699–704.

Harvard Medical Practice Study. *Patients, doctors, and lawyers: Studies of medical injury, malpractice litigation, and patient compensation in New York.* Boston: Harvard Medical Practice Study, 1990, Technical Appendix 5.V.1.

Havas, M., et al. "Provocation study using heart rate variability shows radiation from 2.4 GHz cordless phone affects autonomic nervous system." *European Journal of Oncology* (2010) Library Vol. 5: 273–300.

Heimeier, R.A., et al. "The xenoestrogen bisphenol A inhibits postembryonic vertebrate development by antagonizing gene regulation by thyroid hormone." *Endocrinology* (2009) 150 (6): 2964–2973.

Helm, H.M., et al. "Does private religious activity prolong survival? A six-year follow-up study of 3,851 older adults." *Journals of Gerontology* (2000) 55 (7): M400–M405.

Heneghan, C., et al. "Ongoing problems with metal-on-metal hip implants." *British Medical Journal* (2012) 344: e1349.

Herbstman, J.B., et al. "Prenatal exposure to PBDEs and neurodevelopment." *Environmental Health Perspectives* (2010) 118 (5): 712–719.

Hicks, J.M. "Screening for cancer . . . a very big business." *Healthy Eating Healthy World,* February 21, 2011; accessed January 29, 2013, http://hpjmh.com/2011/02/21/screening-for-cancer-very-big-business/.

———. *Healthy eating healthy world: Unleashing the power of plant-based nutrition.* Dallas: BenBella Books, 2011.

Hippisley-Cox, J., and Coupland, C. "Unintended effects of statins in men and women in England and Wales: Population based cohort study with the QResearch database." *British Medical Journal* (2010) 340: c2197.

Hirzy, J.W., et al. "Comparison of hydrofluorosilicic acid and pharmaceutical sodium fluoride as fluoridating agents: A cost-benefit analysis." *Environmental Science and Policy* (2013) 29: 81–86.

Hobson, K. "CDC: Cancer-screening rates fall short of goals." *Wall Street Journal Health Blog,* January 26, 2012, accessed May 7, 2014, http://blogs.wsj.com/health/2012/01/26/cdc-cancer-screening-rates-fall-short-of-goals/.

Hoffman, J. *HUNZA: Secrets of the world's healthiest and oldest living people.* Clinton, NJ: New Win Publishing, 1997.

———. *Hunza: Ten secrets of the healthiest and oldest living people.* Island Park, NY: Groton, 1968.

Holt-Lunstad, J., et al. "Social relationships and mortality risk: A meta-analytic review." *PLoS Medicine* (2010) 7 (7): e1000316.

Hölzel, B.K., et al. "Mindfulness practice leads to increases in regional brain gray matter density." *Psychiatry Research* (2011) 191 (1): 36–43.

Honig, L.S., et al. "Shorter telomeres are associated with mortality in those with APOE epsilon4 and dementia." *Annals of Neurology* (2006) 60 (2): 181–187.

Horner, J., et al. "Telomerase reactivation reverses tissue degeneration in aged telomerase-deficient mice." *Nature* (2011) 469 (7328): 102–106.

Houston, D.K., et al. "Low 25-hydroxyvitamin D predicts the onset of mobility limitation and disability in community-dwelling older adults: The Health ABC Study." *Journals of Gerontology. Series A, Biological Sciences and Medical Sciences* (2013) 68 (2): 181–187.

———. "Serum 25-hydroxyvitamin D and physical function in adults of advanced age: The CHS All Stars." *Journal of the American Geriatrics Society* (2011) 59 (10): 1793–1801.

Howard, J.M. "Longevity in Hunza land." *Journal of the American Medical Association* (1961) 175 (8): 706.

Huang, X., et al. "Consumption advisories from salmon based on risk of cancer and noncancerous health effects." *Environmental Research* (2006) 101 (2): 263–274.

Hyman, M. "Conventional medicine misunderstands the fundamental laws of biology." drhyman.com, February 16, 2012; accessed January 29, 2013, http://drhyman.com/blog/2012/02/16/conventional-medicine-misunderstands-the-fundamental-laws-of-biology/.

Jacobs, B.S., et al. "Stroke in the young in the Northern Manhattan stroke study." *Stroke* (2002) 33 (12): 2789–2793.

Jacobs, T.L., et al. "Intensive meditation training, immune cell telomerase activity, and psychological mediators." *Psychoneuroendocrinology* (2010) 36 (5): 664–681.

Jain, P., et al. "Commercial soft drinks: pH and *in vitro* dissolution of enamel." *General Dentistry* (2007) 55 (2): 150–154.

Jenkins, D.J.A. "Effect of dietary portfolio of cholesterol-lowering foods given at two levels of intensity of dietary advice on serum lipids in hyperlipidemia: A randomized controlled trial." *Journal of the American Medical Association* (2011) 306 (8): 831–839.

Jensen, B. *Food healing for man.* Escondido, CA: Bernard Jensen, 1983.

Jerschow, E., et al. "Dichlorophenol-containing pesticides and allergies: Results from the US National Health and Nutrition Examination survey 2005–2006." *Annals of Allergy, Asthma and Immunology* (2012) 109 (6): 420–425.

Ju, Y., et al. "Sleep disruption and risk of preclinical Alzheimer's disease." Paper presented at the American Academy of Neurology's 64th annual meeting, New Orleans, February 14, 2012.

Julander, A., et al. "Polybrominated diphenyl ethers—plasma levels and thyroid status of workers at an electronic recycling facility." *International Archives of Occupational and Environmental Health* (2005) 78 (7): 584–592.

Kachuri, L., et al. "Multiple pesticide exposures and the risk of multiple myeloma in Canadian men." *International Journal of Cancer* (2013) 133 (8): 1846–1858.

Kaplan, R.M., and Porzsolt, F. "The natural history of breast cancer." *Archives of Internal Medicine* (2008) 168 (21): 2302–2303.

Karbowski, M., and Neutzner, A. "Neurodegeneration as a consequence of failed mitochondrial maintenance." *Acta Neuropathologica* (2012) 123 (2): 157–171.

Karlamangla, A., et al. "Psychological well-being is positively associated with adult bone mineral density: Findings from the Study of Midlife in the United States." *American Society for Bone and Mineral Research*, October 16, 2012, Abstract MO0316.

Kaslow, A.L., and Miles, R.B. *Freedom from chronic disease.* Los Angeles: Tarcher, 1979.

Kennebeck, J.J. *Why eyeglasses are harmful for children and young people.* New York: Vantage Press, 1969. Available at http://www.i-see.org/eyeglasses_harmful/. Website copy created and edited by Alex Eulenberg, June 2003; last revision November 30, 2003.

Kern, J.K., et al. "Evidence of parallels between mercury intoxication and the brain pathology in autism." *Acta Neurobiologiae Experimentalis* (2012) 72 (2): 113–153.

Klabunde, C.N., et al. "Cancer screening—United States, 2010." *Morbidity and Mortality Weekly Report* (2012) 61 (3): 41–45.

Kleinewietfeld, M., et al. "Sodium chloride drives autoimmune disease by the induction of pathogenic TH17 cells." *Nature* (2013) 496 (7446): 518–522.

Klepac-Ceraj, V., et al. "Relationship between cystic fibrosis respiratory tract bacterial communities and age, genotype, antibiotics, and *Pseudomonas aeruginosa*." *Environmental Microbiology* (2010) 12 (5): 1293–1303.

Kripke, D., et al. "Mortality associated with sleep duration and insomnia." *Archives of General Psychiatry* (2002) 59 (2): 131–136.

Krishnan, N. et al. "Loss of circadian clock accelerates aging in neurodegeneration-prone mutants." *Neurobiology of Disease* (2010) 45 (3): 1129–1135.

Krohn, J. and Taylor, F. *Finding the right treatment*. Point Roberts, WA: Hartley and Marks, 1999.

Lam, V., et al. "Intestinal microbiota determine severity of myocardial infarction in rats." *FASEB Journal* (2012) 26 (4): 1727–1735.

Lanctot, G. *The medical mafia: How to get out of it alive and take back our health and wealth*. Ryde, UK: Bridge of Love Publications, 1995.

Lark, S., and Richards, J. *The chemistry of success*. San Francisco: Bay Books, 2000.

LaRocca, T.J., et al. "Leukocyte telomere length is preserved with aging in endurance exercise-trained adults and related to maximal aerobic capacity." *Mechanisms of Ageing and Development* (2010) 131 (2): 165–167.

LaTuga, M.S., et al. "Beyond bacteria: A study of the enteric microbial consortium in extremely low birth weight infants." *PLoS ONE* (2011) 6 (12): e27858.

Leape, L.L. "Error in medicine." *Journal of the American Medical Association* (1994) 272 (23): 1851–1857.

Lederman, S.A., et al. "Relation between cord blood mercury levels and early child development in a World Trade Center cohort." *Environmental Health Perspectives* (2008) 116 (8): 1085–1091.

Lee, J.R. *Natural progesterone*. Sebastopol, CA: BLL Publishing, 1993.

———. *Optimal health guidelines*. Sebastopol, CA: BLL Publishing, 1993.

Lepp, A., et al. "The relationship between cell phone use, academic performance, anxiety and satisfaction in life in college students." *Computers in Human Behavior* (2014) 31: 343–350.

Levine, Morgan E., et al. "Low protein intake is associated with a major reduction in IGF-1, cancer, and overall mortality in the 65 and younger but not older population." *Cell Metabolism* (2014) 19 (3): 407–417.

Levy, B.R., et al. "Longevity increased by positive self-perceptions of aging." *Journal of Personality and Social Psychology* (2002) 83 (2): 261–270.

Lewontin, R. *Human diversity*. New York: W.H. Freeman, 1982.

Li, D.K., et al. "A population-based prospective cohort study of personal exposure to magnetic fields during pregnancy and the risk of miscarriage." *Epidemiology* (2002) 13 (1): 9–20.

Li, H., et al. "N-nitrosamines are associated with shorter telomere length." *Scandinavian Journal of Work, Environment and Health* (2011) 37 (4): 316–324.

Lin, L., and Li, T.P. "Alteration of telomere length of the peripheral white blood cells in patients with obstructive sleep apnea syndrome." *Journal of Southern Medical University* (2011) 31 (3): 457–460.

Link, A., et al. "Virtual colonoscopy; real misses." *American Journal of Gastroenterology* (2003) 98 (s9): S235.

Linke, A., et al. "Effects of extended-release niacin on lipid profile and adipocyte biology in patients with impaired glucose tolerance." *Atherosclerosis* (2009) 205 (1): 207–213.

Lipski, E. *Digestive wellness*. New Canaan, CT: Keats Publishing, 1996.

Liu, J., et al. "Association of coffee consumption with all-cause and cardiovascular disease mortality." *Mayo Clinic Proceedings* (2013) 88 (10): 1066–1074.

Lowenthal, R.M., et al. "Residential exposure to electric power transmission lines and risk of lymphoproliferative and myeloproliferative disorders: A case-control study." *Internal Medicine Journal* (2007) 37 (9): 614–619.

Luders, E., et al. "Enhanced brain connectivity in long-term meditation practitioners." *NeuroImage* (2011) 57 (4): 1308–1316.

———. "The underlying anatomical correlates of long-term meditation: Larger hippocampal and frontal volumes of gray matter." *NeuroImage* (2009) 45 (3): 672–678.

Lustig, R.H., et al. "The toxic truth about sugar." *Nature* (2012) 482 (7383): 27–29.

Macfarlane, G.T., and Cummings, J.H. "The colonic flora, fermentation, and large bowel digestive function." In *Large intestine: Physiology, pathophysiology, and disease*. S.F. Phillips, J.H. Pemberton, and R.G. Shorter (Eds). San Diego: Raven Press, 1991, pp. 55–72.

Macon, M.B., and Fenton, S.E. "Endocrine disrupters and the breast: Early life effects and later life disease." *Journal of Mammary Gland Biology and Neoplasia* (2013) 18 (1): 43–61.

Malkin, D. "Simian virus 40 and non-Hodgkin lymphoma." *Lancet* (2002) 359 (9309): 812–813.

Masi, S., et al. "Oxidative stress, chronic inflammation, and telomere length in patients with periodontitis." *Free Radical Biology and Medicine* (2011) 50 (6): 730–735.

Masley, S., et al. "Effect of mercury levels and seafood intake on cognitive function in middle-aged adults." *Integrative Medicine* (2012) 11 (3): 32–40.

Mazdai, A., et al. "Polybrominated diphenyl ethers in maternal and fetal blood samples." *Environmental Health Perspectives* (2003) 111 (9): 1249–1252.

McCann, J.C., and Ames, B.N. "Adaptive dysfunction of selenoproteins from the perspective of the triage theory: Why modest selenium deficiency may increase risk of diseases of aging." *FASEB Journal* (2011) 25 (6): 1793–1814.

McCullough, M.E., et al. "Religious involvement and mortality: A meta-analytic review." *Health Psychology* (2000) 19 (3): 211–222.

McDonnell, W.M., and Loura, F. "Complications of colonoscopy." *Annals of Internal Medicine* (2007) 147 (3): 212–213.

McDougall, C. "The men who live forever." *Men's Health*, June 28, 2006.

McGee, C.T. *How to survive modern technology*. New Canaan, CT: Keats Publishing, 1979.

McGowan, K. "Can we cure aging? Controlling inflammation could be the key to a healthy old age." *Discover Magazine*, December 2007; accessed January 29, 2013, http://discovermagazine.com/2007/dec/can-we-cure-aging.

McTaggert, L. *What doctors don't tell you*. San Francisco, CA: Thorsons/Harper Collins, 1996.

Meinig, G. *The root canal cover up*. Ojai, CA: Bion Publishing, 1998.

Mendelsohn, R.S. *Confessions of a medical heretic*. Chicago: Contemporary Books, 1979.

Mertz, J.R., and Wallman, J. "Choroidal retinoic acid synthesis: A possible mediator between refractive error and compensatory eye growth." *Experimental Eye Research* (2000) 70 (4): 519–527.

Meydani, S.N., et al. "Serum zinc and pneumonia in nursing home elderly." *American Journal of Clinical Nutrition* (2007) 86 (4): 1167–1173.

Miehlke, K., et al. *Enzymes: The fountain of life*. Mount Pleasant, SC: Neville Press, 1994.

Mild, K.H., et al. "Pooled analysis of two Swedish case-control studies on the use of mobile and cordless telephones and the risk of brain tumours diagnosed during 1997–2003." *International Journal of Occupational Safety and Ergonomics* (2007) 13 (1): 63–71.

Miller, N.Z., and Goldman, G.S. "Infant mortality rates regressed against number of vaccine doses routinely given: Is there a biochemical or synergistic toxicity?" *Human and Experimental Toxicology* (2011) 30 (9): 1420–1428.

Minot, S., et al. "Rapid evolution of the human gut virome." *Proceedings of the National Academy of Sciences* (2013) 110 (30): 12450–12455.

Möller-Levet, C.S., et al. "Effects of insufficient sleep on circadian rhythmicity and expression amplitude of the human blood transcriptome." *Proceedings of the National Academy of Sciences* (2013) 110 (12): E1132–E1141.

Morgan, L.L., and Philips, G. "Cell phones and brain tumors: 15 reasons for concern," electromagnetichealth.org, August 25, 2009; accessed January 29, 2013, http://electromagnetichealth.org/electromagnetic-health-blog/cellphones-cause-brain-tumors-says-new-report-by-international-emf-collaborative/.

Mostafalou, S., and Abdollahi, M. "Pesticides and human chronic diseases: Evidences, mechanism, and perspectives." *Toxicology and Applied Pharmacology* (2013) 268 (2): 157–177.

Mueller, N.T., et al. "Soft drink and juice consumption and risk of pancreatic cancer: The Singapore Chinese Health Study." *Cancer Epidemiology, Biomarkers and Prevention* (2010) 19 (2): 447–455.

Murphy, L.R. "Stress management in work settings: A critical review of the health effects." *American Journal of Health Promotion* (1996) 11 (2): 112–135.

Murphy, S.L., et al. "Deaths: Preliminary data for 2010." *Division of Vital Statistics, National Vital Statistics Reports* (2012) 60 (4).

Murphy, S.P., et al. "Demographic and economic factors associated with dietary quality for adults in the 1987–88 nationwide Food Consumption Survey." *Journal of the American Dietetic Association* (1992) 92 (11): 1352–1357.

Mutter, J., et al. "Mounting evidence indicates mercury as a specific risk factor for regressive autism." *Neuro Endocrinology Letters* (2005) 26 (5): 439–446.

Naci, H., and Ioannidis, J.P.A. "Comparative effectiveness of exercise and drug interventions on mortality outcomes: Metaepidemiological study." *British Medical Journal* (2013) 347: f5577.

Nataf, R., et al. "Porphyrinuria in childhood autistic disorder: Implications for environmental toxicity." *Toxicology and Applied Pharmacology* (2006) 214 (2): 99–108.

Navarro, E.A., et al. "The microwave syndrome: A preliminary study in Spain." *Electromagnetic Biology and Medicine* (2003) 22 (2–3): 161–169.

Neiman, D.C., et al. "Upper respiratory tract infection is reduced in physically fit and active adults." *British Journal of Sports Medicine* (2011) 45 (12): 987–992.

Nelson, D., et al. "Alcohol-attributable cancer deaths and years of potential life lost in the United States." *American Journal of Public Health* (2013) 103 (4): 641–648.

Nemec, K. "Americans are overmedicating." *Total Health Institute*, April 8, 2012; accessed May 7, 2014, http://www.totalhealthinstitute.com/americans-are-overmedicating/.

Neustadt, J., and Pieczenik, S.R. "Medication-induced mitochondrial damage and disease." *Molecular Nutrition and Food Research* (2008) 52 (7): 780–788.

Newberg, A.B., et al. "Meditation effects on cognitive function and cerebral blood flow in subjects with memory loss: A preliminary study." *Journal of Alzheimer's Disease* (2010) 20 (2): 517–526.

Newman, T.B., and Hully, S. B. "Carcinogenicity of lipid-lowering drugs." *Journal of the American Medical Association* (1996) 275: 55–60.

Ngwezi, D.P., et al. "Congenital heart disease and the emission of industrial development toxicands in Alberta, Canada." *American Heart Association*. Poster Presentation 15332, November 17, 2013.

Nison, P. *The raw life: Becoming natural in an unnatural world.* New York: Three Forty Three, 2000.

Northen, C. "Modern miracle men—Relating to proper food mineral balances." *Cosmopolitan*, June 1, 1936.

Null, G. *Get healthy now.* New York: Seven Stories, 1999.

Null, G., et al. *Death by Medicine.* Edinburg, VA: Axios Press, 2011.

Oberfeld, G., et al. "The microwave syndrome: Further aspects of a Spanish Study." Presented at an international conference in Kos, Greece, May 2004.

Office of Technology Assessment, Congress of the United States. *Assessing the efficacy and safety of medical technologies.* Washington, D.C.: U.S. Government Printing Office, 1978.

Ohnishi, M., et al. "Dietary and genetic evidence for phosphate toxicity accelerating mammalian aging." *FASEB Journal* (2010) 24 (9): 3562–3571.

Okereke, O.I., et al. "High phobic anxiety is related to lower leukocyte telomere length in women." *PLoS ONE* (2012) 7 (7): e40516.

Oman, D., and Reed, D. "Religion and mortality among the community-dwelling elderly." *American Journal of Public Health* (1998) 88 (10): 1469–1475.

Ondicova, K., et al. "The role of the vagus nerve in depression." *Neuro Endocrinology Letters* (2010) 31 (5): 602–608.

Ornstein, R., and Sobel, D. *The healing brain.* New York: Simon and Schuster, 1987.

Oski, F. *Don't drink your milk.* Brushton, NY: TEACH Services, 1983.

Osterholm, M.T., et al. "Efficacy and effectiveness of influenza vaccines: A systematic review and meta-analysis." *Lancet Infectious Diseases* (2012) 12 (1): 36–44.

———. *The compelling need for game-changing influenza vaccines: An analysis of the influenza vaccine enterprise and recommendations for the future.* Center for Infectious Disease Research and Policy, University of Minnesota, October 2012.

Ott, J. *Health and light.* Columbus, OH: Ariel Press, 1976.

Ovelgönne, J.H., et al. "Decreased levels of heat shock proteins in gut epithelial cells after exposure to plant lectins." *Gut* (2000) 46 (5): 679–687.

Oz, M., and Roizen, M. *You: The owner's manual.* New York: William Morrow, 2008.

Pan, A., et al. "Red meat consumption and mortality results from 2 prospective cohort studies." *Archives of Internal Medicine* (2012) 172 (7): 555–563.

Park, M. "Diet cola drains calcium in women." CNNhealth.com, July 7, 2010; accessed January 29, 2013, http://thechart.blogs.cnn.com/2010/07/07/diet-cola-drains-calcium-in-women/.

Patel, S.R., et al. "A prospective study of sleep duration and mortality risk in women." *SLEEP* (2004) 27 (3): 440–444.

Patrick, L. "Thyroid disruption: Mechanism and clinical implications in human health." *Alternative Medicine Review* (2009) 14 (4): 326–346.

Paul, L. "Diet, nutrition, and telomere length." *Journal of Nutritional Biochemistry* (2011) 22 (10): 895–901.

Pauling, L. *How to live longer and feel better.* New York: Avon Books, 1986.

Pearce, J. "Nutrition beliefs: More fashion than fact." *FDA Consumer,* June 1976: 25–27.

Perez-Pozo, S.E., et al. "Excessive fructose intake induces the features of metabolic syndrome in healthy adult men: Role of uric acid in the hypertensive response." *International Journal of Obesity (London)* (2010) 34 (3): 454–461.

Pfeiffer, C. *Mental and elemental nutrients: A physician's guide to nutrition and health care.* New Canaan, CT: Keats Publishing, 1976.

Phillips, E. *Kiss your dentist goodbye.* Austin: Greenleaf Book Group, 2010.

Physicians Committee for Responsible Medicine. "Section three: When is surgery unnecessary?" accessed January 29, 2013, http://www.pcrm.org/research/healthcare-professionals/medicine-curriculum/when-is-surgery-unnecessary.

Pietinen, P., et al. "Intake of fatty acids and risk of coronary heart disease in a cohort of Finnish men: The alpha-tocopherol, beta-carotene cancer prevention study." *American Journal of Epidemiology* (1997) 145 (10): 876–887.

Podevin, N., and du Jardin, P. "Possible consequences of the overlap between the CaMV 35S promoter regions in plant transformation vectors used and the viral gene VI in transgenic plants." *GM Crops and Food* (2012) 3 (4): 296–300.

Poling, D. "Running man passes away: Jim Hammond dies in his sleep at age 95." ValdostaDailyTimes.com, accessed January 29, 2013, http://valdostadailytimes.com/local/x1155937321/Running-man-passes-away.

Pottenger, F.M., Jr. *Pottenger's cats.* La Mesa, CA: Price-Pottenger Nutrition Foundation, 1983.

Pusztai, A., et al. "Antinutritive effects of wheat-germ agglutinin and other N-acetylglucosamine-specific lectins." *British Journal of Nutrition* (1993) 70 (1): 313–321.

Puterman, E., et al. "The power of exercise: Buffering the effect of chronic stress on telomere length." *PLoS ONE* (2010) 5 (5): e10837.

Quillin, P. *Beating cancer with nutrition.* Tulsa, OK: Nutrition Time Press, 1994.

Ramagopalan, S.V. "A ChIP-seq defined genome-wide map of vitamin D receptor binding: Associations with disease and evolution." *Genome Research* (2010) 20 (10): 1352–1360.

Randolph, T., and Moss, R. *An alternative approach to allergies.* New York: Harper and Row, 1980.

Rapp, D. *Our toxic world: A wakeup call.* New Brunswick, NJ: Environmental Research Foundation, 2003.

Reddy, P.H. "Mitochondrial medicine for aging and neurodegenerative diseases." *NeuroMolecular Medicine* (2008) 10 (4): 291–315.

Reddy, P.H., and Reddy, T.P. "Mitochondria as a therapeutic target for aging and neurodegenerative diseases." *Current Alzheimer Research* (2011) 8 (4): 393–409.

Reed, K., et al. "HealthGrades: Hospital quality and clinical excellence study." *Lancet* (1995) 346 (8966): 29–32.

Reffelmann, T., et al. "Low serum magnesium concentrations predict cardiovascular and all-cause mortality." *Atherosclerosis* (2011) 219 (1): 280–284.

Report of the Standing Committee on the Scientific Evaluation of Dietary Reference Intakes and Its Panel on Folate, Other B Vitamins, and Choline, and Subcommittee on Upper Reference Levels of Nutrients, Food and Nutrition Board, Institute of Medicine. *Dietary reference intakes for thiamin, riboflavin, niacin, vitamin B6, folate, vitamin B12, pantothenic acid, biotin, and choline.* Washington, D.C.: National Academy Press, 1998.

Richards, J.B., et al. "Higher serum vitamin D concentrations are associated with longer leukocyte telomere length in women." *American Journal of Clinical Nutrition* (2007) 86 (5): 1420–1425.

Richardson, A.J., et al. "Docosahexaenoic acid for reading, cognition and behavior in children aged 7–9 years: A randomized, controlled trial (The DOLAB Study)." *PLoS ONE* (2012) 7 (9): e43909.

Richardson, T., et al. "Molecular modeling and genetic engineering of milk proteins." In *Advanced dairy chemistry: Proteins*. P.F. Fox (Ed.). London: Elsevier Applied Science, 1992, 545–577.

Robbins, J. *Diet for a new America*. Walpole, NH: Stillpoint Publishing, 1987.

———. *Healthy at 100: The scientifically proven secrets of the world's healthiest and longest lived peoples*. New York: Random House, 2006.

Robinson, M.H. "On sugar and white flour . . . the dangerous twins!" In *A physician's handbook on orthomolecular medicine*. R.J. Williams and D.K. Kalita (Eds.). New York: Pergamon Press, 1977, 24–30.

Rodale, J.I. *The healthy Hunzas*. Emmaus, PA: Rodale Press, 1949.

Rosczyk, H.A., et al. "Neuroinflammation and cognitive function in aged mice following minor surgery." *Experimental Gerontology* (2008) 43 (9): 840–846.

Rose, S. *Lifelines: Biology beyond determinism*. New York: Oxford University Press, 1997.

Ross, S.M., et al. "Neurobehavioral problems following low-level exposure to organophosphate pesticides: A systematic and meta-analytic review." *Critical Reviews in Toxicology* (2013) 43 (1): 21–44.

Rowe, W.J. "Correcting magnesium deficiencies may prolong life." *Clinical Interventions in Aging* (2012) 7: 51–54.

Sacks, F.M., et al. "The effect of pravastatin on coronary events after myocardial infarction in patients with average cholesterol levels." *New England Journal of Medicine* (1996) 335 (14): 1001–1009.

Sadetzki, S., et al. "Cellular phone use and risk of benign and malignant parotid gland tumors: A nationwide case-control study." *American Journal of Epidemiology* (2008) 167 (4): 457–467.

Samitz, G., et al. "Domains of physical activity and all-cause mortality: Systemic review and dose-response meta-analysis of cohort studies." *International Journal of Epidemiology* (2011) 40 (5): 1382–1390.

Samsel, A., and Seneff, S. "Glyphosate's suppression of cytochrome P450 enzymes and amino acid biosynthesis by the gut microbiome: Pathways to modern disease." *Entropy* (2013) 15 (4): 1416–1463.

Sauve, S., et al. "Distribution and antidepressants and their metabolites in brook trout exposed to municipal wastewaters before and after ozone treatment: Evidence of biological effects." *Chemosphere* (2011) 83 (4): 564–571.

Savale, L., et al. "Shortened telomeres in circulating leukocytes of patients with chronic obstructive pulmonary disease." *American Journal of Respiratory and Critical Care Medicine* (2009) 179 (7): 566–571.

Schairer, C., et al. "Menopausal estrogen and estrogen-progestin replacement therapy and breast cancer risk." *Journal of the American Medical Association* (2000) 283 (4): 485–491.

Schantz, S.L., et al. "Impairments of memory and learning in older adults exposed to chlorinated biphenyls via consumption of Great Lakes fish." *Environmental Health Perspectives* (2001) 109 (5): 605.

Scheibner, V. *Vaccination: 100 Years of orthodox research shows that vaccines represent a medical assault on the immune system*. Portland, OR: Co-Creative Designs, 1993.

Schnall, E., et al. "The relationship between religion and cardiovascular outcomes and all-cause mortality in the Women's Health Initiative Observational Study." *Psychology and Health* (201) 25 (2): 249–263.

Schneider, M., et al. *The handbook of self-healing*. New York: Penguin Arkana, 1994.

Schoenthaler, S., et al. "The impact of a low food additive and sucrose diet on academic performance in 803 New York City schools." *International Journal of Biosocial Research* (1986) 8 (2): 185–195.

Schreiber, S.L. "Using the principles of organic chemistry to explore cell biology." *Chemical and Engineering News* (1992) 70 (43): 22–32.

Schroeder, H. *The poisons around us*. New Canaan, CT: Keats Publishing, 1978.

Schulze, M.B., et al. "Sugar-sweetened beverages, weight gain, and incidence of type 2 diabetes in young and middle-aged women." *Journal of the American Medical Association* (2004) 292 (8): 927–934.

Schwartz, J. *It's not what you eat but what eats you*. Berkeley, CA: Celestial Arts, 1988.

Selye, H. *The stress of life*. New York: McGraw-Hill, 1978.

Seralini, G.E., et al. "Long-term toxicity of a Roundup herbicide and a Roundup-tolerant genetically modified maize." *Food and Chemical Toxicology* (2012) 50 (11): 4221–4231.

———. "New analysis of a rat feeding study with genetically modified maize reveals signs of hepatorenal toxicity." *Archives of Environmental Contamination and Toxicology* (2007) 52 (4): 596–602.

Shen, J., et al. "Genetic variation in telomere maintenance genes, telomere length and breast cancer risk." *PLoS ONE* (2012) 7 (9): e44308.

Shivapurkar, N., et al. "Presence of simian virus 40 DNA sequences in human lymphomas." *Lancet* (2002) 359 (9309): 851–852.

Sihvonen, R., et al. "Arthroscopic partial meniscectomy versus sham surgery for a degenerative meniscal tear." *New England Journal of Medicine* (2013) 369 (26): 2515–2524.

Simonton, O.C., et al. *Getting well again.* New York: Bantam, 1978.

Simpopoulos, A.P. "The importance of the ratio of omega-6/omega-3 essential fatty acids." *Biomedicine and Pharmacotherapy* (2002) 56 (8): 365–379.

Singh-Manoux, A., et al. "Timing of onset of cognitive decline: Results from Whitehall II prospective cohort study." *British Medical Journal* (2012) 344: d7622.

Sjodin, A., et al. "Serum concentrations of polybrominated diphenyl ethers (PBDEs) and polybrominated biphenyl (PBB) in the United States population: 2003–2004." *Environmental Science and Technology* (2008) 42 (4): 1377–1384.

Skowronski, D.M., et al. "The number needed to vaccinate to prevent infant pertussis hospitalization and death through parent cocoon immunization." *Clinical Infectious Diseases* (2012) 54 (3): 318–327.

Smith L. *Feed yourself right.* New York: Dell, 1983.

Smith-Bindman, R. "Projected cancer risks from computed tomographic scans performed in the United States, 2007." *Archives of Internal Medicine* (2009) 169 (22): 2071–2077.

Smoak, B.L., et al. "Changes in lipoprotein profiles during intense military training." *Journal of the American College of Nutrition* (1990) 9 (6): 567–572.

Sonneville, K.R., et al. "Vitamin D, calcium, and dairy intakes and stress fractures among female adolescents." *Archives of Pediatrics and Adolescent Medicine* (2012) 166 (7): 595–600.

Steel, K., et al. "Iatrogenic illness on a general medical service at a university hospital." *New England Journal of Medicine* (1981) 304 (11): 638–642.

Stein, R. "Exercise could slow aging of body, study suggests." *Washington Post,* January 28, 2008; accessed January 29, 2013, http://www.washingtonpost.com/wp-dyn/content/article/2008/01/28/AR2008012801873.html.

Steinman, D. *Diet for a poisoned planet.* New York: Random House, 1990.

Steinman, D., and Epstein, S.S. *The safe shoppers bible.* New York: MacMillan, 1995.

Stitt, P.A. *Fighting the food giants.* 2nd ed. Manitowoc, WI: Natural Press, 1981.

Strum, J.W., et al. "Stroke among women, ethnic groups, young adults and children." In *Handbook of clinical neurology.* M. Fisher (ed.). New York: Elsevier, 2009, pp. 337–353.

Sun, Q., et al. "Healthy lifestyle and leukocyte telomere length in U.S. women." *PLoS ONE* (2012) 7 (5): e38374.

Swerdlow, R.H. "Brain aging, Alzheimer's disease, and mitochondria." *Biochimica et Biophysica Acta* (2011) 1812 (12): 1630–1639.

Taira, K., et al. "Sleep health and lifestyle of elderly people in Ogimi, a village of longevity." *Psychiatry and Clinical Neurosciences* (2002) 56 (3): 243–244.

Tesler, E. "Nutrition and eating: Do Americans practice what they preach?" *Food Product Development* (1978) June: 82–86.

Testa, R., et al. "Leukocyte telomere length is associated with complications of Type-2 diabetes mellitus." *Diabetic Medicine* (2011) 28 (11): 1388–1394.

Thany, S.H., et al. "Neurotoxicity of pesticides: Its relationship with neurodegenerative diseases." *Médecine Sciences (Paris)* (2013) 29 (3): 273–278.

The Endocrine Society. "Fructose sugar makes maturing human fat cells fatter, less insulin-sensitive." *News Room,* 2010; accessed September 2, 2014, https://www.endocrine.org/news-room/press-release-archives/2010/fructose sugarmakesmaturing.

Thomas, D. "Mineral depletion in foods over the period 1940 to 1991." *Nutrition Practitioner* (2001) 2 (1): 27–29.

Treas, J., et al. "Chronic exposure to arsenic, estrogen, and their combination causes increased growth and transformation in human prostate epithelial cells potentially by hypermethylation-mediated silencing of MLH1." *Prostate* (2013) 73 (15): 1660–1672.

Trumbo, P., et al. "Dietary reference intakes: Vitamin A, vitamin K, arsenic, boron, chromium, copper, iodine, iron, manganese, molybdenum, nickel, silicon, vanadium, and zinc." *Journal of the American Dietetic Association* (2001) 101 (3): 294–301.

Tucker, K.L., et al. "Colas, but not other carbonated beverages, are associated with low bone mineral density in older women: The Framingham Osteoporosis Study." *American Journal of Clinical Nutrition* (2006) 84 (4): 936–942.

Tudek, B., et al. "Foci of aberrant crypts in the colons of mice and rats exposed to carcinogens associated with food." *Cancer Research* (1989) 49 (5): 1236–1240.

Ulger, Z., et al. "Intra-erythrocyte magnesium levels and their clinical implication in geriatric outpatients." *Journal of Nutrition, Health and Aging* (2010) 14 (10): 810–814.

U.S. Food and Drug Administration. "Follow-up to the June 4, 2008 early communication about the ongoing safety review of tumor necrosis factor (TNF) blockers (marketed as Remicade, Enbrel, Humira, Cimzia, and Simponi)," accessed January 29, 2013, http://www.fda.gov/Drugs/DrugSafety/PostmarketDrugSafety InformationforPatientsandProviders/DrugSafetyInformationforHeathcareProfessionals/ucm174449.htm.

U.S. Office of Technology Assessment. *Assessing the efficacy and safety of medical technologies.* September 1978.

Valentine, T. "Hidden hazards of microwave cooking." *NEXUS Magazine* (1995) 2 (25).

Valero, M.C., et al. "Eccentric exercise facilitates mesenchymal stem cell appearance in skeletal muscle." *PLoS ONE* (2012) 7 (1): e29760

Vallejo, F., et al. "Phenolic compound contents in edible parts of broccoli inflorescences after domestic cooking." *Journal of the Science of Food and Agriculture* (2003) 83 (14): 1511–1516.

Vander, A. *Nutrition, stress, and toxic chemicals: An approach to environmental health controversies.* Ann Arbor: University of Michigan Press, 1981.

Vasquez, A. *Integrative Rheumatology and Inflammation Mastery.* 3rd ed. *Special Edition for Bastyr University 2014.* Seattle: CreateSpace Independent Publishing Platform, 2014.

Vasquez, A. "The clinical importance of vitamin D (cholecalciferol): A paradigm shift with implications for all healthcare providers." *Alternative Therapies in Health and Medicine* (2004) 10 (5): 28–36.

Velicer, C.M., et al. "Antibiotic use in relation to the risk of breast cancer." *Journal of the American Medical Association* (2004) 291 (7): 827–835.

Vendômois, J.S., et al. "A comparison of the effects of three GM corn varieties on mammalian health." *International Journal of Biological Sciences* (2009) 5 (7): 706–726.

Venkatram, S., et al. "Vitamin D deficiency is associated with mortality in the medical intensive care unit." *Critical Care* (2011) 15 (6): R292.

Verdelho, A., et al. "Physical activity prevents progression for cognitive impairment and vascular dementia: Results from the LADIS (Leukaraiosis and Disability) Study." *Stroke* (2012) 43 (12): 3331–3335.

Vernikos, J. *Sitting kills, moving heals.* Fresno, CA: Linden Publishing, 2011.

Vetter, M.L., et al. "What do resident physicians know about nutrition? An evaluation of attitudes, self-perceived proficiency and knowledge." *Journal of the American College of Nutrition* (2008) 27 (2): 287–298.

Vilchez, R.A., et al. "Association between simian virus 40 and non-Hodgkin lymphoma." *Lancet* (2002) 359 (9309): 817–823.

Vinson, J.A., and Bose, P. "Comparative bioavailability of synthetic and natural vitamin C in guinea pigs." *Nutrition Reports International* (1983) 27 (4): 875–880.

Visciano, P., et al. "Polycyclic aromatic hydrocarbons in fresh and cold-smoked Atlantic salmon filets." *Journal of Food Protection* (2006) 69 (5): 1134–1138.

Vithoulkas, G. "Acceptance speech: Right Livelihood Award (Swedish Parliament)." Accessed January 29, 2013, http://www.vithoulkas.com/en/george-vithoulkas/alternative-nobel-prize/2175-swedish-parliament-speech.html.

Walford, R., and Walford, L. *The anti-aging plan: The nutrient-rich, low-calorie way of eating for a longer life—The only diet scientifically proven to extend your health years.* Boston: Da Capo Press, 2005.

Walker, M. *Secrets of long life.* Old Greenwich, CT: Devin-Adair Publishers, 1984.

Waterland, R., et al. "Season of conception in rural Gambia affects DNA methylation at putative human metastable epialleles." *PLoS Genetics* (2010) 6 (12): e1001252.

Werner, C., et al. "Physical exercise prevents cellular senescence in circulating leukocytes and in the vessel wall." *Circulation* (2009) 120 (24): 2438–2447.

Weverling-Rijnsburger, A.W., et al. "Total cholesterol and risk of mortality in the oldest old." *Lancet* (1997) 350 (9085): 1119–1123.

"Whooping Cough Returns to California After Decades of Decline." *PBS Newshour*. PBS. March 16, 2011. Television.

Wikgrenemail, M., et al. "Short telomeres in depression and the general population are associated with a hypocortisolemic state." *Biological Psychiatry* (2012) 71 (4): 294–300.

Willeit, P., et al. "Telomere length and risk of incident cancer and cancer mortality." *Journal of the American Medical Association* (2010) 304 (1): 69–75.

Williams, R.J. *Nutrition against disease*. New York: Bantam, 1971.

———. *The wonderful world within you*. Wichita, KS: Bio-Communications Press, 1977.

Wilson, J.F., et al. "Balancing the risks and benefits of fish consumption." *Annals of Internal Medicine* (2004) 141 (2): 977–980.

Wolkowitz, O.M., et al. "Leukocyte telomere length in major depression: Correlations with chronicity, inflammation and oxidative stress—preliminary findings." *PLoS ONE* (2011) 5 (3): e17837.

Wong, L.S.M., et al. "Renal dysfunction is associated with shorter telomere length in heart failure." *Clinical Research in Cardiology* (2009) 98 (10): 629–634.

Wright, C.J., and Mueller, C.B. "Screening mammography and public health policy: The need for perspective." *Lancet* (1995) 346 (8966): 29–32.

Wu, M.M., et al. "Dose-response relation between arsenic concentration in well water and mortality from cancers and cardiovascular diseases." *American Journal of Epidemiology* (1989) 130 (6): 1123–1132.

Wyshak, G. "Teenaged girls, carbonated beverage consumption, and bone fractures." *Archives of Pediatric and Adolescent Medicine* (2000) 154 (6): 610–613.

Xu, D., et al. "Multivitamin use and telomere length in women." *American Journal of Clinical Nutrition* (2009) 89 (6): 1857–1863.

———. "Homocysteine accelerates endothelial cell senescence." *FEBS Letters* (2000) 470 (1): 20–24.

Yamaguchi, M. "Role of nutritional zinc in the prevention of osteoporosis." *Molecular and Cellular Biochemistry* (2010) 338 (1–2): 241–254.

Yeargin-Allsopp, M., et al. "Prevalence of autism in a US metropolitan area." *Journal of the American Medical Association* (2003) 289 (1): 49–55.

Yudkin, J. *Pure, white and deadly: The problem with sugar*. New York: HarperCollins, 1972.

Zehetner, J., et al. "PVHL is a regulator of glucose metabolism and insulin secretion in pancreatic beta cells." *Genes and Development* (2008) 22: 3135–3146.

Zhang, X., et al. "A mechanism of sulfite neurotoxicity: Direct inhibition of glutamate dehydrogenase." *Journal of Biological Chemistry* (2004) 279 (41): 43035–43045.

Zhang, X.-M., et al. "Initiation and promotion of colonic aberrant crypt foci in rats by 5-hydroxymethyl-2-furaldehyde in thermolyzed sucrose." *Carcinogenesis* (1993) 14 (4): 773–775.

———. "Promotion of aberrant crypt foci and cancer in rat colon by thermolyzed protein." *Journal of the National Cancer Institute* (1992) 84 (13): 1026–1030.

Zhou, T., et al. "Developmental exposure to brominated diphenyl ethers results in thyroid hormone disruption." *Toxicological Science* (2012) 66 (1): 105–116.

Zittermann, A., et al. "Vitamin D deficiency and mortality risk." *Clinical Nutrition* (2012) 95 (1): 91–100.

INDEX

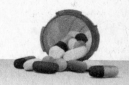